"In this insightful and meticulously researched book, Moorman vividly shows why 'predictable' death is the new American way of death, and elucidates the policies needed to ensure a 'good death' for dying patients and their care providers."

Deborah Carr, *Professor and Chair of Sociology, Boston University*

"This book focuses on the unequal distribution of premature death in contemporary United States. Moorman employs fundamental cause theory to address this vexing problem, providing a compelling discussion to explain differences in health between African Americans and Whites, rich and poor, rural and urban residents and other disadvantaged groups. Her study, grounded in fresh analyses of national data on health and aging trends, comes at a time when understanding complex persistent inequalities in death and dying among the most vulnerable older adults and the potential burden it places on those who care for them, is paramount. With thoughtful new insights and policy prescriptions, *Dying in Old Age: U.S. Practice and Policy* goes beyond sociology and the scholarly research community to inform public officials as well."

Jacqueline Angel, *Professor of Sociology and Public Policy, The University of Texas at Austin*

"Against the backdrop of a comprehensive collection of data and ideas related to trends in contemporary dying, Moorman makes a compelling case for the need (and the means) to adjust our social and health care systems to better serve people at the end of life. An important contribution of her book is the extent to which she documents how people in marginalized groups have been ill-served by our current system."

Mercedes Bern-Klug, *Professor; Director, Aging and Longevity Studies Program, University of Iowa School of Social Work*

DYING IN OLD AGE

Three-quarters of deaths in the U.S. today occur to people over the age of 65, following chronic illness. This new experience of "predictable death" has important consequences for the ways in which societies structure their health care systems, laws, and labor markets. *Dying in Old Age: U.S. Practice and Policy* applies a sociological lens to the end of life, exploring how macrosocial systems and social inequalities interact to affect individual experiences of death in the United States.

Using data from the *National Health and Aging Trends Study* and *Pew Research Center Survey of Aging and Longevity*, this book argues that predictable death influences the entire life course and works to generate greater social disparities. The volume is divided into sections exploring demography, the circumstances of dying people, and public policy affecting dying people and their families. In exploring these interconnected factors, the author also proposes means of making "bad death" an avoidable event.

As one of the first books to explore the social consequences of end of life practice, *Dying in Old Age* will be of great interest to graduate and advanced undergraduate students in sociology, social work, and public health, as well as scholars and policymakers in these areas.

Sara M. Moorman is Associate Professor of Sociology at Boston College, and a fellow of the Gerontological Society of America. In addition to death and dying, Moorman studies life course predictors of cognitive function in older adulthood, as well as psychosocial experiences in older adults' personal relationships.

Society and Aging
Series Editors
Madonna Harrington Meyer, PhD, and
Jennifer Karas Montez, PhD,

Later-Life Social Support and Service Provision in Diverse and Vulnerable Populations
Understanding Networks of Care
Edited by Janet M. Wilmoth and Merril Silverstein

Dying in Old Age
U.S. Practice and Policy
Sara M. Moorman

For a complete list of all books in this series, please visit the series page at: www.routledge.com/Society-and-Aging-Series/book-series/SAS

DYING IN OLD AGE

U.S. Practice and Policy

Sara M. Moorman

Routledge
Taylor & Francis Group
NEW YORK AND LONDON

First published 2021
by Routledge
52 Vanderbilt Avenue, New York, NY 10017

and by Routledge
2 Park Square, Milton Park, Abingdon, Oxon, OX14 4RN

Routledge is an imprint of the Taylor & Francis Group, an informa business

Library of Congress Cataloging-in-Publication Data
A catalog record for this title has been requested

ISBN: 978-1-138-49689-7 (hbk)
ISBN: 978-1-138-49693-4 (pbk)
ISBN: 978-1-351-02018-3 (ebk)

Typeset in Bembo
by Wearset Ltd, Boldon, Tyne and Wear

CONTENTS

TABLES

SERIES EDITOR INTRODUCTION

My father died a good death. It was far too early. He died in his early 60s after a lifetime of smoking a pipe. But he was able to receive at-home hospice care, pain management, and visits with loved-ones until his final breaths. He actively managed his last days, having important conversations, sharing fond memories, and making pivotal decisions about donating his remains for research. It was a death with dignity.

While few people look forward to death, nearly everyone hopes that when the time comes they will die a good death. A death with dignity. But not everyone will.

Good deaths are not randomly distributed. Some people have a much greater chance of dying a good death than others. We think of dying as a fundamentally private, personal event. And yet, it is a fundamentally social, public event as well. A host of social, economic, legal, and political factors shape the quality of our final days and deaths. These structural factors determine who is, and who is not, able to exercise control over the quality of their own dying. This is the topic of Sara M. Moorman's book, *Dying in Old Age: U.S. Policy and Practice.*

She begins by pointing out that the vast majority of the 3 million deaths in the US each year are predictable in that we know the end is near, we can take steps to hasten or postpone final breaths, and we can plan our final days and events. Yet, she cautions, the sociodemographic factors that shape the quality of our lives are the same sociodemographic factors that shape the quality of our deaths, including gender, race, ethnicity, income, education, marital status, geographic location, sexual orientation, and age.

As people approach death, they struggle with managing pain and suffering, finding high-quality care, and feelings of loneliness or social isolation. These struggles feel personal and private but in fact are social and public, shaped by structural factors such as growing inequality, the nature of the US health care system, and our ever-changing laws on advance medical care planning. For example, racial inequality in the US makes it much less likely that Black people will have a good death. Moorman reviews heartbreaking research that shows how Black people are much more likely to be in pain and to receive inadequate pain management, even when controlling for factors such as type of insurance.

Along the way, Moorman addresses hard hitting questions. Do Medicare and Medicaid actually ameliorate or contribute to inequalities in death and dying? Are our advanced medical care laws, sufficient, effective, and manageable, particularly for those with less income, education, and experience? And what about our ever-changing laws concerning passive euthanasia, the practices of refusing and discontinuing treatment near death? Moorman suggests that active euthanasia is the ultimate in predictable death because it permits controlled, managed, assisted deaths. As we go to press, 22% of Americans live in a state in which physician-assisted death was legal at the close of 2019. How do these laws intersect with the inequalities that shape the quality of deaths more generally?

Moorman concludes that we must more fully recognize the social and structural factors that shape the quality of death. She argues that we must also more fully recognize the sociodemographic factors that lead to inequalities in life and inequalities in death. As we reassess and reshape the social, economic, legal, and political structures that shape the quality of death, we have the potential to use them to reduce such inequalities, offering dignity and meaning to all as they approach the end of life.

Madonna Harrington Meyer
University Professor
Syracuse University

1

THE PREDICTABLE DEATH

Each year since 2000, approximately eight of every 1,000 residents of the United States has died (Murphy et al., 2018).[1] In 2018, that amounted to about 3 million people. Someone who is attentive to the news might be excused for believing, for example, that infections with flesh-eating bacteria contribute substantially to that number. But in fact, most deaths in the U.S. today are considerably less newsworthy affairs: Three-quarters of the people who die in the U.S. each year are adults over the age of 65, and they die from one or more chronic illnesses such as heart disease or cancer (Murphy et al., 2018). This regularity or uniformity to death is new, historically speaking, and makes death more *predictable* in at least four ways.

First, deaths today are predictable in that doctors may anticipate them. That is, the major causes of most deaths today are age-related chronic illnesses where the course of illness, the standard treatments, and the general probability of death are well known to medicine (National Center for Health Statistics, 2019). For a variety of reasons discussed in the chapters of this book, doctors may fail to expect a patient's death and may instead experience it as a surprise. An individual's prognosis remains difficult to estimate with much specificity, for example (Christakis, 1999). However, doctors today are 75% accurate at identifying who among their patients is likely to die within the next year (White et al., 2017). This state of affairs is quite different from most of human history, when deaths were unpredictable because they were commonly due to outbreaks of communicable diseases that could afflict persons of any age (Omran, 1971, 1988). Before the invention of vaccines, antibiotics and other drugs, and supportive care techniques, there was comparatively little that medicine could do to prevent death or even to make dying people more comfortable.

Second, today's deaths are predictable because patients have some agency to prevent or delay the major causes of death. Chronic illnesses are sometimes called *lifestyle diseases* because of their strong correlation with diet, exercise, exposure to toxins, and even expectations for the future (Khullar, 2015). Certainly, constraints such as a lack of socioeconomic resources prevent people from being able to live as they might prefer. But people today have a great deal of control over their health compared to the era of communicable diseases, in which people could do little to protect themselves, particularly before the advent of germ theory. Now, for example, adults who say that they expect to live another 50 years take more care with their substance use, sexual risk behavior, exercise frequency, and sleep duration than people who do not expect to survive as long (Scott-Sheldon et al., 2010). Older adults who have a longer personal life expectancy exercise more regularly than people who expect to die at a younger age, and also adhere better to physical therapy regimens aimed at rehabilitation from a disease, injury, or surgery (Kahana et al., 2005; Levy et al., 2012; Ziegelmann et al., 2006). In this way, expectations and desires regarding longevity can be self-fulfilling prophecies now when they could not be ever before (Levy et al., 2002).

Third, death is often predictable enough that people can plan ahead for it, with some scholars arguing that the end of life has become a stage in the life course, like infancy or adolescence (Carr & Luth, 2019). Chronic illnesses are often long enough in duration that people at the end of life may say goodbye to loved ones, write an autobiography, establish legacies, and prepare psychologically or spiritually (Carr, 2012a; Catholic Spiritual Direction, 2015). People can also consider their values and ideas about quality of life, so as to form preferences for medical care in their last days (Carr, 2012b). People can settle their financial affairs: The Federal Trade Commission even provides online tips for savvy shoppers who want to plan their own funerals (Federal Trade Commission, 2012). People may choose not to prepare, or circumstances may prevent them from planning, but this is quite different from a time in which the probability of living to old age was much less certain.

Fourth, because chronic illnesses are long-term and progressive, it is predictable that most people will die in later life after a period – sometimes years – of increasing disability. Governments and societies, as well as individuals and families, need to plan on this period. At the national level, planning includes supporting robust retirement programs for older adults who cannot work as well as creating and staffing health systems to provide universal, ready access to affordable, high-quality health care (Bloom et al., 2015). Local communities need to build and maintain age-friendly infrastructure, such as accessible public transportation, such that people with disabilities can live there (Buffel et al., 2018). These are major economic challenges for the nation, especially given that by mid-century, there will be more Americans over the age of 65 than under the age of 18 (Colby & Ortman, 2014).

About the Book

This book is about predictable death. How did it come about? What social changes made it possible? Now that it is here, what are the unique opportunities it offers and challenges it poses to individuals and societies? How might Americans implement those opportunities and meet the challenges?

In Chapter 2, I explain how, historically, the U.S. arrived at the predictable death. It came about quickly, with increases in life expectancy in the 75 years between 1900 and 1975 that were greater than the increases in the previous 250 years combined (Uhlenberg, 1980). I describe the demography of mortality in 1900, the earliest date for which reliable nationally representative data are available for the United States. I go on to contrast these circumstances with conditions in approximately 2015, along with the substantial effect that increases in death by suicide and overdose had after 2015. I cover epidemiological transition theory, an explanation for these rapid changes.

An emphasis in this book is attention to social inequality. The predictable death involves macrosocial systems that establish patterns of interpersonal experiences at death, which take shape along lines of social difference such as race/ethnicity, social class, gender, marital status, and age. Typically, group inequalities are not neutral; rather, one group suffers the brunt of problems. Usually, members of that group are underrepresented in the institutions that could make effect change, such that their problems are often invisible and obdurate.

Each chapter focuses on one or two sources of stratification. Other inequalities exist, but I do not seek to review them exhaustively in each chapter. Rather, my purpose in drawing focus to different markers in each chapter is to demonstrate the wide array of inequalities in predictable death in the U.S. Chapter 2 focuses on educational attainment and on geographic variation. Educational attainment is associated with disparities in almost all measures of mortality, for every gender and racial/ethnic subgroup, and at all ages (Hummer & Hernandez, 2013). Similarly, where a person lives matters. For example, in 2007, men's life expectancy was higher in 122 other nations than it was in the poorest-faring county in the United States, indicating that far from all Americans enjoy the benefits of living in the wealthiest nation on Earth (Egen et al., 2016). I describe these inequalities and discuss the reasons for their existence and the possibilities for their elimination in the future.

Chapters 3 through 8 address the opportunities and challenges that the predictable death has yielded. I divide these chapters into two three-chapter sections. One of the giants of U.S. sociology, C. Wright Mills (1916–1962), developed in the concept of *private troubles* and *public issues*. His classic example is:

> When, in a city of 100,000, only one man is unemployed, that is his personal trouble, and for its relief we properly look to the character of the man, his skills, and his immediate opportunities. But when in a nation of 50 million employees, 15 million men are unemployed, that is a [public] issue, and we may not hope to find its solution within the range of opportunities open to any one individual.
>
> *(Mills, 1959)*

That is, frequently individuals share their seemingly personal life experiences with others, because those experiences are the product of larger-scale social patterns and historical circumstances.

Chapters 3, 4, and 5 address problems with predictable death that many people regard as intensely intimate and singularly individual: pain and suffering at the end of life, the challenge of finding high-quality care providers for a dying loved one, and the phenomena of loneliness and social isolation. Each chapter illustrates, however, that these problems are remarkably common, even characteristic of, dying in the U.S. today. Far from being the result of individual choices or particular personalities and relationships, these problems are the result of the way the health care economy and the national policies that govern care work and care receipt are structured. These private troubles are in fact public issues of the first order.

Chapter 3 highlights ways in which, ironically, people cannot or do not predict predictable deaths. That is, people generally understand that they will die from their chronic illness, but not when they will die. Half of people who are diagnosed with congestive heart failure, for example, die within five years of diagnosis, while the other half survive more than five years (Mozaffarian et al., 2016). For this and other chronic illnesses, invasive, intensive treatment often becomes the patient's new normal way of life until eventually, treatment fails and he or she dies. Many people go through protracted suffering in an effort to live longer, and death comes as a bit of a surprise. Hospice is one model of an alternative way to approaching dying and death that is more consistent with many people's preferences for their last weeks and days of life. I include suggestions about how doctors, patients, and families could better capitalize on the predictability of death to achieve more comfortable, peaceful deaths.

Racial and ethnic group disparities in experiences at the end of life are the focus of the inequalities segment of Chapter 3. From conception throughout the life course, Americans of color are sicker and more likely to die than White Americans (National Center for Health Statistics, 2016). Thus, when dying, persons of color are more likely than Whites to die in the intensive care unit of a hospital, and less likely than Whites to receive adequate symptoms control and referral to hospice (Johnson, 2013; Tschirhart et al., 2014).

Chapter 4 covers the people whose work is to care for those who die predictable deaths. People who have chronic illnesses often progressively lose independence as they become sicker, which means that they require help with daily tasks. Care work takes place in a variety of settings, including private homes, outpatient clinics, the hospital, and long-term care facilities such as nursing homes and assisted living facilities. Care workers may be paid or unpaid, related to the patient or not. Paid care workers alone comprise 27% of the health care workforce in the United States, and by one estimate, they provide 70 to 80% of the care delivered in long-term care facilities (Dawson, 2016; Harmuth & Dyson, 2005). They constitute one of the largest occupational groups in the United States, outnumbering teachers, cashiers, fast food workers, and public safety workers (PHI, 2011).

One commonality is that both paid and unpaid care workers are typically women whose own socioeconomic status suffers because they provide care: The U.S. has yet to develop viable ways of compensating the people who labor to provide care for people who are dying a predictable death. As a result, older women in poverty in later life are twice as likely to have provided care to their parents compared to older women who have incomes above the poverty line (Wakabayashi & Donato, 2006). Thus one of the sources of stratification I address in this chapter is gender, and the other is nativity. In some states, such as New York and California, immigrants comprise more than 40% of direct care workers, and in some metropolitan areas, such as New York City and Miami, they comprise more than 70% of such workers (Espinoza, 2018; Hess & Henrici, 2013). The vast majority of professional care jobs involve physically and emotionally taxing work for low pay and few benefits, and immigrant women take these jobs because they are unable to get better jobs or lobby for improved conditions within the profession (Hartmann & Hayes, 2017).

Chapter 5 addresses the ways in which loneliness and social isolation are problems for people who are dying predictable deaths. There are fundamental questions about how the predictable death itself – with its concomitant illness and disability – and social isolation mutually generate one another (Holt-Lunstad et al., 2015). Dying people can become lost in cycles of poor physical health, despair, and isolation that did not occur before the predictable death. In keeping with the book's focus on disparities, there is considerable evidence that factors such as old age and poor health, especially poor functional health or disability, place some people at greater risk of social isolation than other people (Garthwaite, 2015).

Chapter 5 is also the chapter in the private troubles section of the book that includes data analysis. I chose two research questions that could be explored in the National Health and Aging Trends Study (NHATS), a longitudinal survey of Medicare beneficiaries. NHATS allows for a novel exploration of several different definitions of social isolation and their relationship to mortality. Very few people are complete recluses with absolutely no connections to others. However, larger numbers of people lack immediate family, or are housebound, or identify as lonely despite whatever social connections they may have. Thus the first research question looks at mortality risk in relation to different ways of being socially isolated. The second research question concerns quality of death. That is, when socially isolated people die – prematurely or otherwise – are their deaths more painful, their quality of care poorer, their wishes less likely to be met? An important element of NHATS is that when participants die, the study team makes every effort to find a family member or health care professional who can report on the decedent's last month of life. Thus, the design elements of NHATS make it quite well-suited for secondary data analysis of these research questions. The chapter works through the analysis step by step, and then interprets the results in light of the strengths and limitations of the data. A data appendix provides additional details for readers who are interested in more exhaustive results or in the statistical methods applied.

Chapters 6, 7, and 8 form the section on public issues. They cover large social systems in the United States, including the Medicare and Medicaid programs, state and federal law, and ethics or morality. These issues are clearly public, both in the sense that they involve government, and in the sense that their operation requires democratic participation. People are often unable to recognize how policy decisions that were made far away by strangers, sometimes decades ago, affect the course of lives in the here and now. Yet they do, and so each chapter goes on to illustrate how dying individuals and their families experience the consequences of these systems as private troubles. For example, a hard decision about a loved one's treatment may seem like the particular result of that person's illness, when in fact the structure of Medicare brings many families around the country to the very same decision point.

Chapter 6 introduces Medicare and Medicaid, the public health insurance programs that cover Americans older than 65 and Americans who require long-term care, respectively. Because Medicare and Medicaid pay many of the health care costs of predictable deaths, they strongly shape families' experiences with predictable death. By paying for some services for dying people and not for others, Medicare and Medicaid incentivize some types of medical care and discourage others. The programs have few benefits that are specific to dying persons, and so the goals that the programs seek for healthier people, such as rehabilitation, are the same goals that they seek for dying people. As a result, two-thirds of decedents are hospitalized in the 6 months before death, and about one-fifth of deaths occur in hospitals (Dartmouth Institute for Health Policy and Clinical Practice, 2019).

These government programs are funded through taxpayer dollars, yet the workings of Medicare and Medicaid are more often bureaucratic decisions rather than democratic ones. Several mechanisms to encourage innovation exist, however, and are bearing fruit. The inequality section of Chapter 6 is about the fruitfulness of Medicare and Medicaid. This section is different from the inequality section of other chapters because in it I address the ways in which these government programs are – and are not – designed to ameliorate social inequalities. Beyond their intent, I also take up the question of whether, in practice, they serve to reduce or exacerbate inequalities.

Chapter 7 explains the U.S. law for advance medical care planning, which is the set of legal mechanisms available to prepare ahead of time for one's own care needs at the end of life. Law has developed somewhat independently of practice, such that advance care plans do not integrate optimally with the ways health care professionals work with dying people and their families. The law aims to promote patient autonomy, while autonomy is only one of several important values that patients and families hold (Ikonomidis & Singer, 1999). Nevertheless, systematic reviews indicate that advance care planning does have a number of benefits, making it a set of laws well worth revision (Brinkman-Stoppelenburg et al., 2014; Khandelwal et al., 2015; Teno et al., 2007).

Chapter 7 addresses social disparities in advance care planning by sexual orientation and by race/ethnicity in advance care planning. U.S. law is organized in large part around the heterosexual married nuclear family, and people who lack that family or are estranged from it find that the advance care planning mechanisms available are largely inapplicable to their situations (Buckey & Browning, 2013). Similarly, persons of color are often either unable to engage in advance care planning due to racism, or reluctant to engage in advance care planning because the available legal mechanisms do not fit the ways they and their loved ones prefer to make health care decisions (Shen et al., 2016).

Chapter 8 concerns euthanasia, which includes both refusing or discontinuing treatment and acting to end life. Euthanasia may be the ultimate in predictable death: controlled, managed, aided. U.S. law on active forms of euthanasia is rapidly changing, with 22% of Americans living in a state in which physician-assisted death was legal at the close of 2019 (Span, 2019). I summarize these changes, as well as data from the U.S. states and European countries that have legalized some forms of active euthanasia. Additionally, I tackle some of the ethical and moral questions that inform law and practice. What are the circumstances in which a person may end his or her own life? Are there any circumstances in which another person may assist a dying person who wants to end his or her life? Social inequalities inform many people's answers to these questions: What disparities might accompany legalization of physician-assisted death or euthanasia?

Chapter 8 is also the chapter in the public issues section of the book that includes data analysis. I chose to explore public opinion in the Pew Research Center's 2013 Survey of Aging and Longevity. Americans' attitudes about the moral acceptability of ending one's own life, and even about assisting someone else in ending their life, have changed rather rapidly over several short decades. In 1990, for example, 27% of the American public agreed that there is "a moral right to suicide when a person is ready to die because living has become a burden." By 2013, 38% of the American public agreed with this statement (Pew Research Center, 2013). Although at a population level, attitudes about euthanasia have become more accepting, these issues remain extremely contentious. For example, the American public is almost evenly split on whether physicians should be able to prescribe a lethal dose of medication with the intention that a terminally ill person take that dose in order to die (i.e., physician-assisted death) (Pew Research Center, 2013). I center the analysis on racial/ethnic differences in public opinion, because of the racial and ethnic disparities in health care throughout the life course. Perhaps as a result of these disparities, Americans of color are much less likely to support euthanasia in several forms, as this analysis and others reveal.

Finally, Chapter 9 concludes the book. I reach three conclusions about predictable death. One is that more people should acknowledge and recognize that death has become predictable, so as to take advantage of the opportunity to plan that it can afford. One is a caution about social disparities: Left alone, predictable death will produce wider and wider inequalities between Americans. Last is that predictable death is a public issue, such that political and civic involvement can help maximize its benefits and minimize its problems. Only public engagement with these issues in a healthy democratic society will curb disparities in who can and cannot realize the opportunities of predictable death.

Frameworks for Conceptualizing Predictable Death

Two theoretical frameworks, the life course perspective and fundamental cause theory, have informed my thinking in this book. The life course perspective is a way of thinking about how individual lives are situated in historical time (Elder et al., 2003). In this case, the lives – and deaths – of people today may be quite different from the lives people of the past were able to realize because today, humans have unprecedented control over death. That control affects the plans people make in their work and family lives, the ways they think about mortality and human purpose, and types of experiences that are normative or unusual. For example, medical anthropologist Sharon Kaufman has written extensively about the medicalization of death, where people today no longer think of death as natural and inevitable, but instead think of it as a medical condition to be managed and prevented as long as possible (Kaufman, 2005).

In addition to a focus on historical time, the life course perspective has a focus on geographical place. The way predictable deaths occur in the U.S. differs somewhat from how predictable deaths occur in other Western nations. For example, legal euthanasia in places such as Belgium and the Netherlands may make death as predictable as it can possibly be (Emanuel et al., 2016). Even within the United States, there are large regional differences in individuals' experiences of health and death because of variation in the composition of the population, differences in environmental conditions, and dissimilar social policies (Kulkarni et al., 2011). A person's risk of dying from opioid overdose, for example, depends a great deal on where they live (Monnat et al., 2019).

However, the life course perspective does not view time and place as deterministic. Within the constraints of government, the economy, and other large-scale social forces, individuals have agency (Hitlin & Elder, 2007). The word's meaning is not a simple "placeholder for some vague sense of human freedom or individual volition;" rather, agency refers to the reflexive relationship between large-scale social forces and the self (Hitlin & Elder, 2007, p. 171). That is, even apparently monolithic structures like the health care system are the product of individuals making choices, and could be remade differently.

Another aspect of agency within the life course perspective is timing. Individuals may have more or less agency depending on when an event or transition takes place. For example, timing of diagnosis with a chronic illness such as cancer has important consequences for the extent to which the disease is treatable and even curable (World Health Organization, 2017). Moreover, timing affects a person's life course in a variety of additional ways. The timing of predictable death in older adulthood, for example, has made early deaths unusual and thus difficult to cope with. For example, one thing that makes a widowed person's grief more bearable is the presence of peers who share the same experience (Balkwell, 1985). People who are widowed at a young age often feel isolated because they lack peers who have had that experience, which may be one reason that widowhood is a risk factor for suicide among younger, but not older, adults (Luoma & Pearson, 2002).

This example highlights the importance of timing, and also the importance of linked lives. The concept of linked lives simply draws attention to the ways in which lives are not independent. One's well-being may depend on the life or death of one's spouse, for example. Further, the burden of grief in people's lives is not equal: Black Americans experience more immediate family deaths, starting earlier in the life course, than White Americans do (Umberson et al., 2017). Thus Black children are at greater risk than White children of having a parent die, for example, an experience with far-reaching consequences throughout the life course (Høeg et al., 2019).

In addition to the life course perspective, fundamental cause theory helps make sense of social disparities in predictable death. Fundamental cause theory begins from the observation that there have been social disparities in health and death throughout recorded history, despite dramatic changes in life expectancy and the major causes of death (Clouston et al., 2016). The factors that produce these disadvantages are known as fundamental causes, meaning that they are resources that have long enabled people to prevent disease and enhance physical safety, regardless of the contemporary conditions that cause illness and death (Link & Phelan, 1995). Originally, fundamental cause theory focused on "knowledge, money, power, prestige, and beneficial social connections," but recently it has expanded to include racism, sexism, and other social stigma as fundamental causes (Hatzenbuehler et al., 2013; Masters et al., 2015; Phelan & Link, 2015, p. 27). The essential features of a fundamental cause are that it represents a flexible resource that can be used to affect multiple risk factors for multiple causes of death enduringly over historical time (Phelan et al., 2010). Resources may be at the individual level, such as personal income, or at the contextual level, such as neighborhood wealth.

Fundamental cause theory describes why, even as efforts in public health and social policy close disparities in old risk factors and causes of death, new risk factors and causes of death move in and replicate the disparities (Miech et al., 2011). For example, infectious diseases such as tuberculosis disproportionately affected poor people. However, reducing the incidence of infectious disease did not successfully eliminate the disparity in mortality between rich and poor people, because the chronic causes of death that replaced infectious disease, such as heart disease, *also* disproportionately affected poor people. Fundamental causes are resources that people can always use to protect their health, regardless of the particular risks they face in daily life and the causes of death they aim to avoid. Thus, people with resources can take advantage of aspects of the predictable death like the time to plan, while also minimizing the problems associated with predictable death, such as the ability to find and afford high-quality long-term care.

In fact, public health and social policy can unwittingly make inequalities stronger because they activate fundamental causes. That is, if little is known about the risk factors for and treatment of a given disease, then people cannot effectively use their resources to prevent or cure it. Once causes are known and publicized, then they are under human control (Oster, 2018). Disparities increase to the extent that causes of death are under human control, because people who have advantages such as high-educational attainment have greater power to exercise control over their health than do disadvantaged people (Phelan & Link, 2005). Thus, the predictable death has brought about new and increasing disparities in health and mortality.

The relationship between socioeconomic status and high cholesterol is an illustrative example (Chang & Lauderdale, 2009). High cholesterol is asymptomatic, but strongly associated with heart disease. Cholesterol levels are partly due to genetics, but are also due to diet, exercise, and smoking. In the U.S. in the 1960s and 1970s, people of high socioeconomic status had higher cholesterol than people of low-socioeconomic status. Advantaged people could afford to purchase and consume high-cholesterol foods, such as red meat and cream. At that time meats and dairy were considered to be very healthy foods, and moreover, there were no effective drug treatments to lower cholesterol. Then, nutrition science uncovered the risks of high-cholesterol diets. A class of drugs called statins was developed in the 1980s, and statins are credited with much of the declines in heart disease mortality. Subsequently, the association between socioeconomic status and high-cholesterol reversed. Wealthier, more educated people are now more likely to have low cholesterol because they (a) visit the doctor and discover that their cholesterol is high, (b) learn about and make the sorts of behavioral changes that lower cholesterol, and (c) obtain, fill, and take prescriptions for statin medications. Conversely, poorer, less educated people may be unaware that their cholesterol is high, unable to afford low-cholesterol diets and find time for exercise, and unaware of or unable to afford medications to treat high cholesterol.

Other good examples of fundamental causes at work are parental income, education, and race/ethnicity in the case of the human papillomavirus (HPV) vaccine and cervical cancer (Polonijo & Carpiano, 2013); regional educational attainment and poverty levels in the case of cigarette smoking and lung cancer (Rubin et al., 2014); race, class, and health insurance access in the case of diabetes management (Lutfey & Freese, 2005); and regional education and poverty in the case of adoption of various advances in controlling heart disease and colon cancer (Phelan & Link, 2005). Additionally, several studies have examined a range of causes of death and concluded that disparities are stronger among more preventable causes than among less preventable causes (Masters et al., 2015; Phelan et al., 2004). Thus, empirical evidence supports the major tenets of fundamental cause theory.

An important development in fundamental cause theory is the idea of countervailing mechanisms (Lutfey & Freese, 2005; Phelan et al., 2010). In the original formulation of the theory, scholars assumed that people are always rational actors who will use their resources to improve their health. But for some people in some circumstances, there are goals more important than health and longevity, the pursuit of which requires dedication of resources in ways that damage health. Key among these is status attainment. For example, people may be willing to risk their health if long, stressful, sedentary hours at work benefit their career. Research is just beginning to describe cases in which advantaged people knowingly deploy their resources for outcomes inconsistent with good health.

Thus, the main points of the life course perspective and fundamental cause theory will make clearer the reasons behind both the advantages and the disadvantages of predictable death. For example, the next chapter illustrates how historically, just as human agency began to matter more for health and mortality, disparities widened because people had differing levels of ability to affect change in their circumstances. These disparities mean that while some people benefit from predictable death, others suffer regardless of the predictability of mortality.

Note

1. This book focuses on death and dying in the United States. Other parts of the world have predictable deaths; indeed, there is a lot to be learned from other places such as the Netherlands, where euthanasia is legal; the U.K., where the health care system is public; and Japan, where the probability of living to be 100 is greater than anywhere else in the world. However, U.S. state and federal law, U.S. programs such as Medicare and Medicaid, and U.S. policy on institutional and family caregiving are just three factors that profoundly shape death and dying in the U.S. context.

References

Balkwell, C. (1985). An attitudinal correlate of the timing of a major life event: The case of morale in widowhood. *Family Relations*, *34*(4), 577–581. https://doi.org/10.2307/584022.

Bloom, D. E., Canning, D., & Lubet, A. (2015). Global population aging: Facts, challenges, solutions & perspectives. *Daedalus*, *144*(2), 80–92. https://doi.org/10.1162/DAED_a_00332.

Brinkman-Stoppelenburg, A., Rietjens, J. A., & van der Heide, A. (2014). The effects of advance care planning on end-of-life care: A systematic review. *Palliative Medicine*, *28*(8), 1000–1025. https://doi.org/10.1177/0269216314526272.

Buckey, J. W., & Browning, C. N. (2013). Factors affecting the LGBT population when choosing a surrogate decision maker. *Journal of Social Service Research*, *39*(2), 233–252. https://doi.org/10.1080/01488376.2012.754205.

Buffel, T., Handler, S., & Phillipson, C. (2018). *Age-friendly cities and communities: A global perspective*. Policy Press.

Carr, D. (2012a). Death and dying in the contemporary United States: What are the psychological implications of anticipated death? *Social and Personality Psychology Compass*, *6*(2), 184–195. https://doi.org/10.1111/j.1751-9004.2011.00416.x.

Carr, D. (2012b). "I don't want to die like that . . .": The impact of significant others' death quality on advance care planning. *The Gerontologist, 52*(6), 770–781. https://doi.org/10.1093/geront/gns051.

Carr, D., & Luth, E. A. (2019). Well-being at the end of life. *Annual Review of Sociology, 45*(1), 515–534. https://doi.org/10.1146/annurev-soc-073018-022524.

Catholic Spiritual Direction. (2015). *Preparation for death*. https://spiritualdirection.com/topics/meditations/preparation-for-death.

Chang, V. W., & Lauderdale, D. S. (2009). Fundamental cause theory, technological innovation, and health disparities: The case of cholesterol in the era of statins. *Journal of Health and Social Behavior, 50*(3), 245–260. https://doi.org/10.1177/002214650905000301.

Christakis, N. A. (1999). *Death foretold*. University of Chicago Press.

Clouston, S. A. P., Rubin, M. S., Phelan, J. C., & Link, B. G. (2016). A social history of disease: Contextualizing the rise and fall of social inequalities in cause-specific mortality. *Demography, 53*(5), 1631–1656. https://doi.org/10.1007/s13524-016-0495-5.

Colby, S. L., & Ortman, J. M. (2014). *The Baby Boom cohort in the United States: 2012 to 2060* (No. P25-1141; Current Population Reports). United States Census Bureau. www.census.gov/content/dam/Census/library/publications/2014/demo/p25-1141.pdf.

Dartmouth Institute for Health Policy and Clinical Practice. (2019). *Dartmouth atlas of health care*. www.dartmouthatlas.org/data/table.aspx?ind=15.

Dawson, S. L. (2016). The direct care workforce – Raising the floor of job quality. *Generations, 40*(1), 38–46.

Egen, O., Beatty, K., Blackley, D. J., Brown, K., & Wykoff, R. (2016). Health and social conditions of the poorest versus wealthiest counties in the United States. *American Journal of Public Health, 107*(1), 130–135. https://doi.org/10.2105/AJPH.2016.303515.

Elder, G. H., Johnson, M. K., & Crosnoe, R. (2003). The emergence and development of life course theory. In J. T. Mortimer & M. J. Shanahan (Eds.), *Handbook of the life course* (pp. 3–19). Springer US. https://doi.org/10.1007/978-0-306-48247-2_1.

Emanuel, E. J., Onwuteaka-Philipsen, B. D., Urwin, J. W., & Cohen, J. (2016). Attitudes and practices of euthanasia and physician-assisted suicide in the United States, Canada, and Europe. *Journal of the American Medical Association, 316*(1), 79–90. https://doi.org/10.1001/jama.2016.8499.

Espinoza, R. (2018). *Immigrants and the direct care workforce*. PHI. https://phinational.org/resource/immigrants-and-the-direct-care-workforce-2018/.

Federal Trade Commission. (2012). *Shopping for funeral services*. www.consumer.ftc.gov/articles/0070-shopping-funeral-services.

Garthwaite, K. (2015). "Keeping meself to meself" – How social networks can influence narratives of stigma and identity for long-term sickness benefits recipients. *Social Policy & Administration, 49*(2), 199–212. https://doi.org/10.1111/spol.12119.

Harmuth, S., & Dyson, S. (2005). *Results of the 2005 national survey of state initiatives on the long-term care direct-care workforce*. National Clearinghouse on the Direct Care Workforce. https://phinational.org/wp-content/uploads/legacy/clearinghouse/RESULTS%20OF%20THE%202005%20NATIONAL%20SURVEY%20FINAL%2092205.pdf.

Hartmann, H., & Hayes, J. (2017). The growing need for home care workers: Improving a low-paid, female-dominated occupation and the conditions of its immigrant workers. *Public Policy & Aging Report, 27*(3), 88–95. https://doi.org/10.1093/ppar/prx017.

Hatzenbuehler, M. L., Phelan, J. C., & Link, B. G. (2013). Stigma as a fundamental cause of population health inequalities. *American Journal of Public Health, 103*(5), 813–821. https://doi.org/10.2105/AJPH.2012.301069.

Hess, C., & Henrici, J. M. (2013). *Increasing pathways to legal status for immigrant in-home care workers*. Institute for Women's Policy Research. https://iwpr.org/publications/increasing-pathways-to-legal-status-for-immigrant-in-home-care-workers/.

Hitlin, S., & Elder, G. H. (2007). Time, self, and the curiously abstract concept of agency. *Sociological Theory, 25*(2), 170–191. https://doi.org/10.1111/j.1467-9558.2007.00303.x.

Høeg, B. L., Johansen, C., Christensen, J., Frederiksen, K., Dalton, S. O., Bøge, P., Dencker, A., Dyregrov, A., & Bidstrup, P. E. (2019). Does losing a parent early influence the education you obtain? A nationwide cohort study in Denmark. *Journal of Public Health, 41*(2), 296–304. https://doi.org/10.1093/pubmed/fdy070.

Holt-Lunstad, J., Smith, T. B., Baker, M., Harris, T., & Stephenson, D. (2015). Loneliness and social isolation as risk factors for mortality: A meta-analytic review. *Perspectives on Psychological Science, 10*(2), 227–237. https://doi.org/10.1177/1745691614568352.

Hummer, R. A., & Hernandez, E. M. (2013). The effect of educational attainment on adult mortality in the United States. *Population Bulletin, 68*(1), 1–16.

Ikonomidis, S., & Singer, P. A. (1999). Autonomy, liberalism and advance care planning. *Journal of Medical Ethics, 25*(6), 522–527. https://doi.org/10.1136/jme.25.6.522.

Johnson, K. S. (2013). Racial and ethnic disparities in palliative care. *Journal of Palliative Medicine, 16*(11), 1329–1334. https://doi.org/10.1089/jpm.2013.9468.

Kahana, E., Kahana, B., & Zhang, J. (2005). Motivational antecedents of preventive proactivity in late life: Linking future orientation and exercise. *Motivation and Emotion, 29*(4), 438–459. https://doi.org/10.1007/s11031-006-9012-2.

Kaufman, S. R. (2005). *… And a time to die*. University of Chicago Press.

Khandelwal, N., Kross, E. K., Engelberg, R. A., Coe, N. B., Long, A. C., & Curtis, J. R. (2015). Estimating the effect of palliative care interventions and advance care planning on ICU utilization: A systematic review. *Critical Care Medicine, 43*(5), 1102–1111. https://doi.org/10.1097/CCM.0000000000000852.

Khullar, D. (2015). Reducing lifestyle diseases means changing our environment. *Scientific American*. https://blogs.scientificamerican.com/guest-blog/reducing-lifestyle-diseases-means-changing-our-environment/.

Kulkarni, S. C., Levin-Rector, A., Ezzati, M., & Murray, C. J. (2011). Falling behind: Life expectancy in U.S. counties from 2000 to 2007 in an international context. *Population Health* Metrics, 9, 16. https://doi.org/10.1186/1478-7954-9-16.

Levy, B. R., Slade, M. D., Kunkel, S. R., & Kasl, S. V. (2002). Longevity increased by positive self-perceptions of aging. *Journal of Personality and Social Psychology, 83*(2), 261–270. https://doi.org/10.1037//0022-3514.83.2.261

Levy, B. R., Slade, M. D., Murphy, T. E., & Gill, T. M. (2012). Association between positive age stereotypes and recovery from disability in older persons. *Journal of the American Medical Association, 308*(19), 1972–1973. https://doi.org/10.1001/jama.2012.14541.

Link, B. G., & Phelan, J. (1995). Social conditions as fundamental causes of disease. *Journal of Health and Social Behavior*, 80–94. https://doi.org/10.2307/2626958.

Luoma, J. B., & Pearson, J. L. (2002). Suicide and marital status in the United States, 1991–1996: Is widowhood a risk factor? *American Journal of Public Health, 92*(9), 1518–1522. https://doi.org/10.2105/AJPH.92.9.1518.

Lutfey, K., & Freese, J. (2005). Toward some fundamentals of fundamental causality: Socioeconomic status and health in the routine clinic visit for diabetes. *American Journal of Sociology, 110*(5), 1326–1372. https://doi.org/10.1086/428914.

Masters, R. K., Link, B. G., & Phelan, J. C. (2015). Trends in education gradients of 'preventable' mortality: A test of fundamental cause theory. *Social Science & Medicine, 127*, 19–28. https://doi.org/10.1016/j.socscimed.2014.10.023.

Miech, R., Pampel, F., Kim, J., & Rogers, R. G. (2011). The enduring association between education and mortality: The role of widening and narrowing disparities. *American Sociological Review, 76*(6), 913–934. https://doi.org/10.1177/0003122411411276.

Mills, C. W. (1959). *The sociological imagination*. Oxford University Press.

Monnat, S. M., Peters, D. J., Berg, M. T., & Hochstetler, A. (2019). Using Census data to understand county-level differences in overall drug mortality and opioid-related mortality by opioid type. *American Journal of Public Health, 109*(8), 1084–1091. https://doi.org/10.2105/AJPH.2019.305136.

Mozaffarian, D., J., B. E., Go Alan S., Arnett Donna K., Blaha Michael J., Cushman Mary, Das Sandeep R., de Ferranti Sarah, Després Jean-Pierre, Fullerton Heather J., Howard Virginia J., Huffman Mark D., Isasi Carmen R., Jiménez Monik C., Judd Suzanne E., Kissela Brett M., Lichtman Judith H., Lisabeth Lynda D., Liu Simin, … Turner Melanie B. (2016). Heart disease and stroke statistics – 2016 update. *Circulation, 133*(4), e38–e360. https://doi.org/10.1161/CIR.0000000000000350.

Murphy, S. L., Xu, J., Kochanek, K., & Arias, E. (2018). *Mortality in the United States, 2017* (NCHS Data Brief No. 328). National Center for Health Statistics. www.cdc.gov/nchs/products/databriefs/db328.htm.

National Center for Health Statistics. (2016). *Health, United States, 2015*. www.ncbi.nlm.nih.gov/books/NBK367640/.

National Center for Health Statistics. (2019). *10 leading causes of death by age group, United States 2017*. www.cdc.gov/injury/images/lc-charts/leading_causes_of_death_by_age_group_2017_1100w850h.jpg.

Omran, A. R. (1971). The epidemiologic transition: A theory of the epidemiology of population change. *The Milbank Quarterly, 49*(4), 509–538. https://doi.org/10.1111/j.1468-0009.2005.00398.x.

Omran, A. R. (1988). The epidemiologic transition theory revisited thirty years later. *World Health Statistics Quarterly, 51*(2–4), 99–119.

Oster, E. (2018). *Behavioral feedback: Do individual choices influence scientific results?* [National Bureau of Economic Research Working Paper]. National Bureau of Economic Research. https://doi.org/10.3386/w25225.

Pew Research Center. (2013). *Views on end-of-life medical treatments*. www.pewforum.org/2013/11/21/views-on-end-of-life-medical-treatments/.

Phelan, J. C., & Link, B. G. (2005). Controlling disease and creating disparities: A fundamental cause perspective. *The Journals of Gerontology: Series B, 60*(Special_Issue_2), S27–S33. https://doi.org/10.1093/geronb/60.Special_Issue_2.S27.

Phelan, J. C., & Link, B. G. (2015). Is racism a fundamental cause of inequalities in health? *Annual Review of Sociology, 41*(1), 311–330. https://doi.org/10.1146/annurev-soc-073014-112305.

Phelan, J. C., Link, B. G., Diez-Roux, A., Kawachi, I., & Levin, B. (2004). "Fundamental causes" of social inequalities in mortality: A test of the theory. *Journal of Health and Social Behavior, 45*(3), 265–285. https://doi.org/10.1177/002214650404500303.

Phelan, J. C., Link, B. G., & Tehranifar, P. (2010). Social conditions as fundamental causes of health inequalities: Theory, evidence, and policy implications. *Journal of Health and Social Behavior, 51*(1_suppl), S28–S40. https://doi.org/10.1177/0022146510383498.

PHI. (2011). *Who are direct-care workers?* https://phinational.org/wp-content/uploads/legacy/clearinghouse/PHI%20Facts%203.pdf.

Polonijo, A. N., & Carpiano, R. M. (2013). Social inequalities in adolescent human papillomavirus (HPV) vaccination: A test of fundamental cause theory. *Social Science & Medicine, 82*, 115–125. https://doi.org/10.1016/j.socscimed.2012.12.020.

Rubin, M. S., Clouston, S., & Link, B. G. (2014). A fundamental cause approach to the study of disparities in lung cancer and pancreatic cancer mortality in the United States. *Social Science & Medicine, 100*, 54–61. https://doi.org/10.1016/j.socscimed.2013.10.026.

Scott-Sheldon, L., Carey, M. P., Vanable, P. A., & Senn, T. E. (2010). Subjective life expectancy and health behaviors among STD clinic patients. *American Journal of Health Behavior, 34*(3), 349–361. https://doi.org/10.5993/AJHB.34.3.10.

Shen, M. J., Prigerson, H. G., Paulk, E., Trevino, K. M., Penedo, F. J., Tergas, A. I., Epstein, A. S., Neugut, A. I., & Maciejewski, P. K. (2016). Impact of end-of-life discussions on the reduction of Latino/non-Latino disparities in do-not-resuscitate order completion. *Cancer, 122*(11), 1749–1756. https://doi.org/10.1002/cncr.29973.

Span, P. (2019, July 8). Aid in dying soon will be available to more Americans. Few will choose it. *New York Times*. www.nytimes.com/2019/07/08/health/aid-in-dying-states.html.

Teno, J. M., Gruneir, A., Schwartz, Z., Nanda, A., & Wetle, T. (2007). Association between advance directives and quality of end-of-life care: A national study. *Journal of the American Geriatrics Society, 55*(2), 189–194. https://doi.org/10.1111/j.1532-5415.2007.01045.x.

Tschirhart, E. C., Du, Q., & Kelley, A. S. (2014). Factors influencing the use of intensive procedures at the end of life. *Journal of the American Geriatrics Society, 62*(11), 2088–2094. https://doi.org/10.1111/jgs.13104.

Uhlenberg, P. (1980). Death and the family. *Journal of Family History, 5*(3), 313–320. https://doi.org/10.1177/036319908000500304.

Umberson, D., Olson, J. S., Crosnoe, R., Liu, H., Pudrovska, T., & Donnelly, R. (2017). Death of family members as an overlooked source of racial disadvantage in the United States. *Proceedings of the National Academy of Sciences, 114*(5), 915–920. https://doi.org/10.1073/pnas.1605599114.

Wakabayashi, C., & Donato, K. M. (2006). Does caregiving increase poverty among women in later life? Evidence from the Health and Retirement survey. *Journal of Health and Social Behavior, 47*(3), 258–274. https://doi.org/10.1177/002214650604700305.

White, N., Kupeli, N., Vickerstaff, V., & Stone, P. (2017). How accurate is the 'surprise question' at identifying patients at the end of life? A systematic review and meta-analysis. *BMC Medicine, 15*(1), 1–14. https://doi.org/10.1186/s12916-017-0907-4.

World Health Organization. (2017). *Guide to early cancer diagnosis*. http://apps.who.int/iris/bitstream/10665/254500/1/9789241511940-eng.pdf.

Ziegelmann, J. P., Lippke, S., & Schwarzer, R. (2006). Subjective residual life expectancy in health self-regulation. *The Journals of Gerontology: Series B, 61*(4), P195–P201. https://doi.org/10.1093/geronb/61.4.P195.

2

THE DEMOGRAPHY OF DEATH

This chapter explains how death became predictable in the U.S. and elsewhere. Before approximately 1900, many lives were indeed "nasty, brutish, and short," as Thomas Hobbes famously stated (Hobbes, 1886, p. 64). Child death was ordinary, and death for people of any age was usually the result of sudden violent illness. Subsequently, the entire world has seen dramatic increases in the length of lifetimes since 1900, such that 2% of Americans will live 100 years or more (Arias et al., 2017). Many deaths are predictable: illnesses respond to medicine and to individual health behaviors, and people can plan for their needs before and after death. Demographers call the large changes that occurred in this period the *epidemiologic transition*, and I explain how this theory accounts for the changes. However, there remains a great deal of inequality across the globe, and even across the U.S., in who is able to enjoy a predictable death, or avoid the problems it has caused. Differences across the population in both educational attainment and geography are associated with inequalities in mortality. I show those disparities and illustrate the reasons why they persist.

The United States in 1900

Life expectancy at birth in the U.S. in 1900 was only 47 years.[1] Just as an average test grade in a class represents both students who earned As and students who earned Ds, life expectancy at birth represents both people who will live to be very old and people who will die in infancy or childhood. Thus, although the average person could expect to die at 47, there was considerable variation around this mean and the high probability of death in infancy contributed heavily to the low average. Infancy was perilous, and one out of every ten newborns died (Centers for Disease Control and Prevention, 1999). However, 41% of people born in 1900 lived to be 65 and 14% lived to be 80, so later life did exist as a normative stage in the life course for some (Arias et al., 2017).

People tended to fall ill rather suddenly and die quickly from contagious illnesses such as pneumonia or influenza, tuberculosis, and gastrointestinal infections (D. S. Jones et al., 2012). These diseases spread quickly in cities, which had many people living in close quarters and often, using dirty water (Condran & Crimmins, 1980). As they still are today, the very young and the very old were particularly at risk of dying from these diseases. Half of all parents experienced the death of a child under the age of 15, and only a quarter of newborns had 4 living grandparents (Uhlenberg, 1980).

Around the world, conditions varied greatly in 1900. Life expectancy in Canada, the United Kingdom, Western Europe, and Japan was similar to life expectancy in the United States, between 45 and 50 years (Roser, 2019). Leading causes of death in these places were also similar (Johansson & Mosk, 1987). Yet conditions were much poorer in the rest of the world: Life expectancy was only 23 in India, and 25 in Mexico. Much of the world was highly susceptible to famine, and to epidemics of diseases such as plague and influenza (McAlpin, 1983).

The United States in the 21st Century

By 2014, U.S. newborns were much safer than in 1900, with fewer than six babies dying per thousand births (Centers for Disease Control and Prevention, 1999). These dramatic decreases in infant mortality drove an average life expectancy that rose to 79 years (Arias et al., 2017). Eighty-four percent of those born in 2014 are expected to live to be 65 and 58% will live to be 80 (Arias et al., 2017). Though still rare, living to be 100 is more common than at any other time in history. Since 1980, the number of U.S. centenarians increased 66%, compared to the population as a whole, which increased 36% (Meyer, 2012). Recent decades have even seen centenarians and near-centenarians fit enough to complete marathons (Iqbal, 2011). Human biologists do not, however, believe that life expectancy will ever reach 100 years (Carnes et al., 2013). Rather, they estimate that societies would need to eliminate *all* preventable mortality, including accidents and injuries, for life expectancy to even reach 90 years.

The improvements in life expectancy between 1900 and 2014 were unprecedented in human history. The increases in life expectancy in the 75 years between 1900 and 1975 alone were greater than the increases in the 250 years between and 1650 and 1900 (Uhlenberg, 1980). However, 2015, 2016, and 2017 saw small declines in U.S. life expectancy – to 78.6 years in 2017 – when no decline had occurred since the 1960s (Murphy et al., 2018). Deaths among younger adults, largely due to overdoses of opioid pain medication, accounted for the decline (Khazan, 2017). Overall, *deaths of despair* from suicide, drug overdose, or liver disease related to alcohol abuse have risen among rural White non-Hispanic people who have less than a high-school education, likely due to increased poverty and unemployment (Peters et al., 2019; Scutchfield & Keck, 2017).

While life expectancy increased, variation around the mean life expectancy decreased, making death ever more predictable. Demographers use the term *compression of mortality* to describe the hypothetical scenario in which there is no variability around average life expectancy. That is, mortality is maximally "compressed" if average life expectancy is 76 years and everyone dies on their 76th birthday. In the U.S. today, much of the variation in age at death among younger decedents has been eliminated: Approximately three-quarters of deaths happen to people over the age of 65 (Engelman et al., 2010). There continues to be room to further compress mortality among older decedents, because although most deaths have been postponed into older adulthood, various sociodemographic inequalities mean that the most advantaged people still live longest. Some scholars believe that compression of mortality will continue as healthier people age into later life, although economic inequalities among children and youth are growing and may halt further compression of mortality (Currie & Schwandt, 2016; Warren, 2016).

Causes of the Epidemiologic Transition

Just as life expectancy has increased since 1900, the major causes of death have shifted as well. Since 1975, the top two causes of death after have been cancer and heart disease (National Center for Health Statistics, 2017). Stroke was the third leading cause until the mid-2000s, and is now the fourth behind chronic lower respiratory diseases such as emphysema (National Center for Health Statistics, 2018). Alzheimer's disease ranks 6th overall, and 5th among people over the age of 65. These are non-communicable diseases that occur mostly among older people and kill over a matter of years rather than days. The risk factors are elements of lifestyle: smoking, unhealthy diet (and relatedly, high cholesterol), physical inactivity, and high blood pressure (Bauer et al., 2014). Further, even the death rates from cancer, heart disease, and stroke have been decreasing since 1969, because advances in prevention and treatment have increased the duration of time that people survive with these illnesses (Ma et al., 2015). This epidemiologic transition from death at a young age from infectious disease to death in old age from chronic conditions has occurred all over the world, albeit at varying rates (Omran, 1971, 1988).

Initially, scholars attributed these changes to economic modernity; that is, to improved standards of living (McKeown & Brown, 1955). These scholars did not believe that advances in medicine, such as vaccinations, and advances in public health, such as water filtration, were sufficiently powerful to explain the transition. Instead, they thought that increased economic well-being allowed people to choose an overall healthier lifestyle, in particular a more nutritious diet, which in turn enhanced the body's resistance to infectious disease (McKeown, 1976, 1979).

This position implied that health was subject to broad economic forces, while direct health interventions had little effect on population health. This view held considerable sway with the U.S. government in the mid-1970s and early 1980s, as it suggested that accelerations in the market economy would improve health without any need for the state to intervene by investing public money in medicine and public health (Szreter, 2002). This view also dovetailed nicely with conservative political movements of the time that emphasized personal responsibility. That is, individuals were responsible for engaging in a healthy lifestyle and were to blame for diseases caused by their own unhealthy choices (Knowles, 1977).

However, the position that broad improvements in the economy, rather than direct health interventions, explained historical declines in mortality was not entirely true (Johansson, 1994; Szreter, 1988). What is true is that the relatively crude curative treatments available in the early 1900s had little effect (Colgrove, 2002). Nevertheless, broad public health initiatives and improved knowledge about domestic hygiene did play a major role in increasing life expectancy. Water filtration and chlorination systems were installed in U.S. cities during the first decades of the 1900s, and were responsible for dramatic mortality reductions, especially among infants and young children (Cutler & Miller, 2005). Germ theory began to receive attention in the popular press, and mechanisms of household ventilation, redesigned toilets, and disinfectants for household use exploded commercially (Tomes, 1990). Vaccine development and U.S. immunization policy reduced mortality from diseases such as diphtheria, measles, and mumps by 100% since peaks in the 1930s through the 1950s (Roush et al., 2007). Standards for the clean production of cow's milk, pasteurization processes, and regulations on the quality of milk for retail sale also contributed to greater survival for infants and children (Lee, 2007).

Important initiatives continued to reduce mortality in the mid to late-1900s, including safe antibiotic drugs, the introduction of Medicaid and Medicare, enforced speed limits on roads, and improved treatment for cardiovascular disease (Crimmins, 1981). In recent decades, within infant and child mortality near zero, improvements in survival have primarily been due to reductions in later life mortality. These reductions are due to decreased tobacco use among men and, for both genders, even better treatments for cardiovascular disease (Mathers et al., 2015). Various innovations in public health and medicine have certainly improved the health of the population (Zheng & George, 2018).

However, public health alone is insufficient to explain all of the epidemiologic transition (Condran & Crimmins-Gardner, 1978). There continues to be debate about the extent of the role that economic development, particularly the industrial revolution, played in the epidemiologic transition. By one estimate, increases in per capita income account for 15% of increases in life expectancy through approximately 1975 (Preston, 1975).[2] Undoubtedly, standards of living improved dramatically at the same time as life expectancy increased rapidly. But two empirical findings limit scholars' enthusiasm for considering economic development to be a major cause of life expectancy increases. First, the industrial revolution had been underway for some time before declines in mortality began (Easterlin, 2000). In fact, the rise of polluted, crowded industrial cities probably worked to significantly counteract life expectancy benefits from higher income (Easterlin, 1999; Granados, 2005). Second, mortality has declined across the globe, while economic development has not had similar universal gains. Cutler and colleagues (2006) give the example that people in China in the year 2000 had a per capita income that was similar to the U.S. in 1870, paired with a life expectancy that was similar to the U.S. in 1970. If economic modernity and life expectancy were closely coupled, then life expectancy would not be as high as it is in many low-income nations. Nevertheless, public health certainly requires economic development: Economic development creates institutional capacity, without which nations cannot engage in public health initiatives (Cutler et al., 2006).

The unfortunate enduring legacy of the public health vs. economic modernity debate is that it created a competition: Should the government invest in life expectancy directly through health initiatives, or should it investing indirectly by changing broader socioeconomic policies (Frenk & Gómez-Dantés, 2017)? Ultimately, both economic development and public health produced the epidemiologic transition. Continued improvements in life expectancy will depend on the institutions and individuals that control economic resources choosing to use their power in ways that enhance population health (Woolf & Braveman, 2011).

Educational Disparities in Mortality

In this section, I focus on educational attainment, which is associated with disparities in health and mortality however they are measured, for every gender and racial/ethnic subgroup, and at all ages (Hummer & Hernandez, 2013). For example, a 2012 article in *Health Affairs* authored by a large team of prominent gerontologists received a great deal of media attention (Olshansky et al., 2012). One of their most striking estimates was that in 2008, life expectancy for White men with a college degree was 14 years longer than life expectancy for Black men who had not completed high school. Such differences, the gerontologists asserted, made life in the U.S. so unequal that it was more like two nations than one. Life expectancy figures that aggregate all people in the U.S. obscure large social disparities.

This article drew significant attention to an issue that researchers had been documenting since the early 1990s: Already sizeable educational disparities in life expectancy had been growing (Kitagawa & Hauser, 1973; Preston & Elo, 1995). Each year of primary and secondary school reduces adults' mortality risk, which drops dramatically among high-school graduates, and then continues to decline for each year of education past high school (Montez et al., 2012).

Subsequently, researchers directed their attention towards the group of adults who do not complete high school. However, this association is complex, given that average educational attainment increased at the same time that educational disparities in mortality grew. Women and members of some racial/ethnic groups, in particular, made gains in educational attainment (Everett et al., 2011). Failing to graduate high school is increasingly unusual, such that the population of adults who do not have a high-school diploma is increasingly small and select. This phenomenon makes life expectancy appear to be dropping among people who fail to graduate from high school, when in fact it is remaining stable (Bound et al., 2015). In fact, the primary source of increasing disparity is increasing life expectancy among the most highly educated Americans (Hayward et al., 2015; Ma et al., 2012; Montez et al., 2011). For example, people who hold a high-school diploma have mortality rates that are 80% higher than those of people who hold a professional degree (Rogers et al., 2010).

Educational attainment is related not only to life expectancy, but also to variation in life expectancy, that is, compression of mortality. Mortality is most compressed among people with the highest levels of education (Brown et al., 2012; Sasson, 2016). Highly educated people have lower overall rates of disease than do less educated people, and they also experience later ages of onset when they do become sick (Dupre, 2007, 2008).

There are two key questions to answer about these disparities. The first is why the disparity exists; that is, how does education allow people to live longer? The second is why the disparity has been expanding. That is, why does education have greater longevity benefits than it did in the past?

Education is a fundamental cause of health disparities. It affects life expectancy through several mechanisms that are extremely complex, despite the apparent simplicity of measuring years of education (Elo, 2009). Indeed, Hummer and Hernandez (2013) note that we know almost nothing about some of the most complex and difficult-to-measure dimensions of education that are surely important, such as the content of the curriculum and the quality of instruction. Nor do we know much about how age of school attendance and completion, for example, college at the age of 18–22 versus college as a returning adult learner, matter for health (Walsemann et al., 2018). With these considerable gaps in mind, I address the relationships between years of education and health behaviors, between years of education and access to other resources, and between years of education and cognitive ability and learned effectiveness.

First, education teaches people health literacy, or the skills and abilities to understand and use new information about health (Nutbeam, 2008). Highly educated people are the first to learn about new innovations in medicine, and about health behaviors that will risk, maintain, or improve their health (Oster, 2018). For example, more highly educated people are less likely to take up cigarette smoking, as well as more likely to quit smoking if they are already smokers (Denney et al., 2010). Alcohol consumption and physical inactivity also differ greatly between people who have little education and people who have more (Nandi et al., 2014). Accordingly, deaths from causes that can be the result of health behaviors, such as cardiovascular disease, injury, and overdose, are much less common among highly educated people than among those who have less education (McKenzie et al., 2012; Sasson, 2016).

Second, education enables people to accumulate other resources in adulthood, such as high income. The correlation between educational attainment and income is at a historical high (Hout, 2012). Income inequality has been increasing in the United States since the 1970s, such that annual income among the lowest-earning 20% of Americans was $25,600 or less in 2018, while annual income among the highest-earning 20% of Americans was $130,000 or more (Semega et al., 2019). Inequality itself is a cause of poor health within societies (Pickett & Wilkinson, 2015). Consequences are especially dire for low-income people. For example, costs to attend a public college rose 31% in the decade between 2007 and 2017, putting educational attainment increasingly out of reach for many families (National Center for Education Statistics, 2019). Those low and middle-income families that do send their children to college face debt, with one-third of Americans under 30 having outstanding student loans, which average $25,000 (Houle, 2014; Pew Research Center, 2019).

In addition to income, people with higher educational attainment have better access to health insurance and high-quality health care, prestigious jobs that are physically safe, and supportive social networks. These aspects of socioeconomic status cluster together, accounting for some of the effects of educational attainment on mortality (Montez & Barnes, 2016). Indeed, other evidence suggests that education is less salubrious when it co-occurs with other social disadvantages, such as among people of color (Fuller-Rowell et al., 2015). There is debate over whether education can serve to compensate for early life adversities, with some studies concluding that it can (Schafer et al., 2013), and other studies concluding that it cannot (Montez & Hayward, 2014). Zajacova (2012; Zajacova & Everett, 2014) has documented that high-school dropouts who eventually complete a General Equivalency Diploma (GED) do not realize the same health benefits as students who complete traditional high school, further indicating that social risk factors can limit the benefits of education.

Third, education confers learned effectiveness, a sense of control over and agency in one's own life (Mirowsky & Ross, 2003). Part of learned effectiveness is the development of abstract, higher-order cognitive skills, such that educated people are experienced problem-solvers, risk-assessors, and decision-makers (Baker et al., 2011; Herd, 2010). Another part of learned effectiveness is non-cognitive skills such as self-confidence, planfulness, and ability to cooperate with others (D. E. Jones et al., 2015). Together, the cognitive and non-cognitive skills learned in school allow individuals to obtain and maintain good health and live longer.

However, these three explanations for the link between education and mortality do not shed light on why educational disparities in mortality have increased over the past several decades. Increases are due in part to cohort replacement: As members of older, more homogeneous cohorts die, they are replaced with members of younger, more diverse cohorts, such that the disparity in the population as a whole increases. The educational disparity in mortality is larger for younger cohorts, such as the Millennials, than it is for older cohorts, such as the Baby Boomers (Masters et al., 2012).

The reason that younger cohorts have larger educational disparities in mortality, and the second reason why the educational disparity in mortality has increased, is that the major causes of death have changed across cohorts (Masters et al., 2015). Educational attainment affects emerging major causes of death, such as opioid overdose, even more strongly than it affected past major causes of death, such as lung cancer (Miech et al., 2011). Reductions in smoking greatly decreased the incidence of lung cancer, but could not entirely eliminate it because lung cancer has additional causes that are less controllable (Pampel et al., 2015). In contrast, death by opioid overdose is entirely preventable.

This literature suggests that education policy in childhood, adolescence, and young adulthood is health policy for later life. Inequality begins early in life, and investments in education produce returns, decades later, in higher life expectancy and increasingly compressed mortality (Chaudry et al., 2017). Education not only yields tangible benefits such as job skills, but also prevents disease and other undesirable social outcomes (e.g., crime). Similar to other efforts at prevention in public health, education is much less expensive than treating ill health once it has already developed (Heckman, 2006; Thornton et al., 2016). However, society has been moving in the opposite direction: Inequality in childhood has been increasing for decades, and government policies have not ameliorated it (Western et al., 2008; Woolf & Braveman, 2011). These trends will almost certainly result in health disparities when those children reach adulthood (Hayward & Gorman, 2004; Warren, 2016).

Geographic Disparities in Mortality

In addition to disparities in mortality by educational attainment, there are sweeping geographical disparities in mortality. In broad scale, people in the U.S. are very advantaged compared to people in other parts of the world. Sub-Saharan Africa fares particularly poorly: In 2015, life expectancy in Sierra Leone was only 50 and in Angola, it was only 52 (World Health Organization, 2016). Life expectancy was higher in these places until the 1990s, when the HIV/AIDS epidemic struck Africa and began to lower life expectancy. In 2016, over a quarter of the population in both Swaziland and Lesotho was infected with HIV (World Bank, 2019). The majority of new HIV infections continue to occur in Africa, where many infants are infected during pregnancy and birth (U.S. Department of Health & Human Services, 2018).

However, the U.S. no longer compares as well as it once did to other parts of the world. The World Health Organization estimated that in 2015, 30 countries had a higher life expectancy than the U.S. (World Health Organization, 2016). These included New Zealand and Australia, Canada, Singapore and Korea, Chile, and most European nations. The highest life expectancy in the world was Japan, at 83.7 years. Experts in social epidemiology observe that most other high-income nations have more expansive and generous social policies at all stages of the life course, including universal health care, comprehensive early childhood education, and employment protection, than the United States does (Avendano & Kawachi, 2014). The U.S. also has comparatively high levels of income and wealth inequality (Santacreu & Zhu, 2017), and social inequality is itself a cause of poor health (Pickett & Wilkinson, 2015).

Although international differences in life expectancy are dramatic, most inequality is due to factors within countries (Smits & Monden, 2009). There are major geographic inequalities in survival within the United States, on a scale that nations such as Japan, the United Kingdom, and Canada do not experience. For example, life expectancy for U.S. men in 2007 was 76 years, but this varied across counties from 66 years in Holmes County, Mississippi to 81 years in Fairfax County, Virginia, a difference of over 15 years (Kulkarni et al., 2011). Men's life expectancy was higher in 122 other nations than it was in the poorest-faring county in the United States, indicating that far from all Americans enjoy the benefits of living in a high-income country (Egen et al., 2016).

Inequalities are evident across many different scales of analysis. At a broad scale, there is a great deal of research on the rural–urban divide in life expectancy. Before the advent of water sanitation practices and other major public health initiatives, rural areas were healthier than urban areas. But by 1969, urban life expectancy was about five months longer than rural life expectancy (Singh & Siahpush, 2014). That gap has expanded: In 2009, urban life expectancy was 79 years, and rural life expectancy was almost two and a half years shorter (Singh & Siahpush, 2014). Just as life expectancy in general is sensitive to infant and child deaths, such deaths have an outsized influence on the rural–urban disparity. For example, in 2013, infant mortality was 16% higher in the rural Appalachian region of the country than it was elsewhere (Singh et al., 2017).

However, the rural–urban divide is not simple. The most rural areas – with a population of fewer than 2,500 people and not adjacent to a metropolitan area – do not differ in life expectancy from urban areas (James, 2014). These healthy rural areas are predominantly in the upper Midwest. It is rural areas with a population between 2,500 and 19,999 that are adjacent to metropolitan areas, which are especially common in the South, that fare worst (James, 2014). The reason is that rurality seems to compound other health disparities, such that the lowest rural mortality rates for Blacks remain higher than the highest rural mortality rates for White non-Hispanic people (James & Cossman, 2017).

At a slightly smaller scale, there are regional and state-level disparities in mortality. Overall, life expectancy is lowest in the Southeastern U.S. and highest in the coastal Northeast, the upper Midwest, and coastal California (Kulkarni et al., 2011). The four leading causes of death – cancer, stroke, heart disease, and chronic lower respiratory disease – all demonstrate this disparity. For example, cancer patients are most likely to die in Kentucky, Arkansas, and Mississippi, and least likely to die in Arizona, Utah, and Colorado (Mokdad et al., 2017). Seven states in the Southeast are known as the Stroke Belt, where stroke incidence and mortality are markedly higher than elsewhere in the U.S. Even people who lived in the Stroke Belt in childhood and subsequently moved elsewhere have an increased risk of stroke (Glymour et al., 2007). Heart disease mortality (Gillum et al., 2012) and chronic lower respiratory disease mortality (Holt et al., 2011) are both worst in the Southeast, as well.

There remain distinct disparities in mortality at some of the smallest geographic scales. For example, the Bay Area Rapid Transit (BART) system conveniently connects parts of coastal California. Life expectancy at birth in the community at the Walnut Creek BART stop was 84 years in 2013, compared with 73 years in the Oakland City Center community just 16 miles away (Choi, 2013). The Robert Wood Johnson Foundation and Virginia Commonwealth University have mapped similar discrepancies in major metropolitan areas across the United States, as well as in smaller, less affluent cities such as Tulsa, Oklahoma (Robert Wood Johnson Foundation, 2015; Virginia Commonwealth University Center on Society and Health, 2016).

Such variation has multiple causes. One is compositional differences, where people with lower or higher life expectancies due to other disparities also live together in certain places. For example, 58% of Blacks in the U.S. live in the South (Office of Minority Health, 2019). But perhaps the most encompassing answer to why there are geographic differences in health and mortality is that differences in social policies, which respond in part to the composition of the population, produce different sets of resources and problems on the ground. I discuss three such outcomes of public policy, as they vary across geographic place, here: local environmental risks, level of health care access, and degree of state control over health policy.

First, human well-being depends on the earth's well-being, and some physical and natural environments are safer and more conducive to health than others. For example, the Southeast U.S., which is already behind the rest of the country in life expectancy, is also especially susceptible to the sea level rise, hurricanes, droughts, and heat waves that are consequences of climate change. In addition to the physical danger and the possibility of losing one's house and livelihood in natural disasters, these changes also bring such health risks as increased incidence of foodborne illness, polluted water supplies, and diseases carried by mosquitoes and ticks (Gutierrez & LePrevost, 2016). Moreover, in the long term, wealth inequality increases in places that have experienced natural disasters, as a consequence of the policies by which disaster insurance programs reimburse residents (Howell & Elliott, 2019)

Compounding environmental problems is the not-in-my-backyard phenomenon, whereby wealthy people have the political clout to keep manmade hazards out of their neighborhoods. Thus unhealthy neighborhoods, such as those near noisy, dirty highways, airports, and train lines, are disproportionately the residences of poor people and people of color (Stuart et al., 2009). Most businesses are uninterested in investing in these neighborhoods, and so it is difficult for residents to purchase healthy food (Zenk et al., 2015) and easy for them to purchase alcohol (Bluthenthal et al., 2008). Alcohol availability increases rates of violent crime, which means that residents are hesitant to venture outdoors to exercise (Gómez et al., 2004; Gorman et al., 2001). This example illustrates how neighborhoods rarely have a single health risk, but rather experience an accumulating cascade of environmental and social risks.

A second, well-studied cause of geographic differences in health and mortality is access to high-quality health care. There are several dimensions to this problem. One is the simple presence or absence of facilities in an area. Mortality rates are higher the farther that people have to travel to reach health care facilities (Yamashita & Kunkel, 2010). Rural areas, in particular, tend to lack health care providers (Bolin et al., 2015; Fields et al., 2016). A second dimension is the availability of high-quality care facilities in an area. Many facilities are understaffed, overcrowded, and lack the resources necessary to deliver quality care. People of color tend to be segregated near, or be routed to, low-quality sources of care (Dimick et al., 2013; Khera et al., 2015). A third dimension is individuals' ability to afford treatment, regardless of whether they have nearby health facilities and regardless of the overall quality of the facilities where they receive treatment. People who lack consistent health insurance have poorer health than people who can afford regular and preventive care (Spencer et al., 2013). Health insurance is geographically patterned: Inconsistent health insurance is a particular barrier to care for rural dwellers (Fields et al., 2015).

Finally, Montez (2017; Montez et al., 2017) argues compellingly that three broad policy changes – deregulation, devolution, and pre-emption – have produced large state-level variations in public health policy, and thus in mortality and survival, since 1980. *Deregulation* refers to reduced government oversight of private industry and business. For example, the government has an interest in regulating products that contribute to the obesity epidemic. In response, the food and beverage industry has lobbied against government regulations, and argued that it is able and willing to regulate itself (Nixon et al., 2015).

The other two terms describe a consolidation of power at the state level. *Devolution* describes decreases in the power of the federal government relative to state governments. For example, devolution has increased state-to-state variation in services available through Medicaid. Mortality declined significantly in New York, Maine, and Arizona, three states that adopted Medicaid expansions in the early 2000s, as compared to Pennsylvania, New Hampshire, Nevada, and New Mexico, neighboring states that did not expand the program (Sommers et al., 2012). Other research links mortality differences to state-level tobacco control policies and cigarette prices (Polednak, 2011). Tobacco-growing states have been slow to adopt the types of policies that have decreased tobacco-related mortality in other states (Fallin & Glantz, 2015).

Finally, *pre-emption* describes policies that have served to increase the power of the state government relative to local governments. Pre-emption prevents municipalities from making their own public health laws that differ from state law (Pertschuk, Pomeranz, et al., 2013; Pomeranz & Pertschuk, 2017). Pre-emption policies have limited the efficacy of local movements concerning a range of public health issues, from tobacco control in Oklahoma (Douglas et al., 2015) to residential fire sprinklers in Texas (Pertschuk, Hobart, et al., 2013), to alcohol licensing and control in New York (Mosher & Treffers, 2013).

Summary

This chapter has described the sociohistorical processes that have led to the predictable death. The epidemiological transition was the nation's move from death at early ages from infectious causes to death at increasingly older ages from non-communicable diseases. The epidemiological transition has occurred – or is in the process of occurring – across the world, and is the result of both general economic development and investment in medicine and public health. However, serious inequalities in length and quality of life remain. Educational attainment is one major factor in inequalities in mortality, where Americans who obtain the highest levels of education are enjoying ever longer, healthier lives. Education confers health literacy and learned effectiveness, as well as material resources such as wealth and social connections. Thus, policies that affect education have secondary effects on health and mortality. Policies, including but not limited to health policies, also produce large geographic disparities in mortality. Policies affect the level of local environmental risk, the accessibility of health care resources, and even the degree to which other policies vary across space. Deregulation, devolution, and pre-emption are important processes that have reduced government control overall and solidified remaining government control at the state level.

Notes

1. Life expectancy differs from life span, which is the number of years a creature actually lives. Record life spans are difficult to verify given questions of accuracy in record-keeping in the distant past, but Jeanne Calment, who died at the age of 122, remains the widely accepted record holder (Daley, 2019). The maximum length of the life span for humans as a species is still actively debated, but is currently estimated at approximately 115 years (Gavrilova & Gavrilov, 2019).
2. There are no later estimates available.

References

Arias, E., Heron, M., & Xu, J. (2017). *United States life tables, 2014* (No. 66–4; National Vital Statistics Reports). National Center for Health Statistics. www.cdc.gov/nchs/data/nvsr/nvsr66/nvsr66_04.pdf.

Avendano, M., & Kawachi, I. (2014). Why do Americans have shorter life expectancy and worse health than do people in other high-income countries? *Annual Review of Public Health*, *35*(1), 307–325. https://doi.org/10.1146/annurev-publhealth-032013-182411.

Baker, D. P., Leon, J., Smith Greenaway, E. G., Collins, J., & Movit, M. (2011). The education effect on population health: A reassessment. *Population and Development Review*, *37*(2), 307–332. https://doi.org/10.1111/j.1728-4457.2011.00412.x.

Bauer, U. E., Briss, P. A., Goodman, R. A., & Bowman, B. A. (2014). Prevention of chronic disease in the 21st century: Elimination of the leading preventable causes of premature death and disability in the USA. *The Lancet*, *384*(9937), 45–52. https://doi.org/10.1016/S0140-6736(14)60648-6.

Bluthenthal, R. N., Cohen, D. A., Farley, T. A., Scribner, R., Beighley, C., Schonlau, M., & Robinson, P. L. (2008). Alcohol availability and neighborhood characteristics in Los Angeles, California and Southern Louisiana. *Journal of Urban Health*, *85*(2), 191–205. https://doi.org/10.1007/s11524-008-9255-1.

Bolin, J. N., Bellamy, G. R., Ferdinand, A. O., Vuong, A. M., Kash, B. A., Schulze, A., & Helduser, J. W. (2015). Rural healthy people 2020: New decade, same challenges. *The Journal of Rural Health*, *31*(3), 326–333. https://doi.org/10.1111/jrh.12116.

Bound, J., Geronimus, A. T., Rodriguez, J. M., & Waidmann, T. A. (2015). Measuring recent apparent declines in longevity: The role of increasing educational attainment. *Health Affairs*, *34*(12), 2167–2173. https://doi.org/10.1377/hlthaff.2015.0481.

Brown, D. C., Hayward, M. D., Montez, J. K., Hummer, R. A., Chiu, C.-T., & Hidajat, M. M. (2012). The significance of education for mortality compression in the United States. *Demography*, *49*(3), 819–840. https://doi.org/10.1007/s13524-012-0104-1.

Carnes, B. A., Olshansky, S. J., & Hayflick, L. (2013). Can human biology allow most of us to become centenarians? *The Journals of Gerontology: Series A*, *68*(2), 136–142. https://doi.org/10.1093/gerona/gls142.

Centers for Disease Control and Prevention. (1999). Achievements in public health, 1900–1999: Healthier mothers and babies. *Morbidity and Mortality Weekly Report*, *48*(38), 849–858.

Chaudry, A., Morrissey, T., Weiland, C., & Yoshikawa, H. (2017). *Cradle to kindergarten: A new plan to combat inequality*. Russell Sage Foundation.

Choi, L. (2013). *Health and wealth inequities across Bay Area Rapid Transit (BART) stations*. Federal Reserve Bank of San Francisco. www.frbsf.org/community-development/blog/health-wealth-inequality-bay-area-bart/.

Colgrove, J. (2002). The McKeown thesis: A historical controversy and its enduring influence. *American Journal of Public Health*, *92*(5), 725–729. https://doi.org/10.2105/AJPH.92.5.725.

Condran, G. A., & Crimmins, E. (1980). Mortality differentials between rural and urban areas of states in the northeastern United States 1890–1900. *Journal of Historical Geography*, *6*(2), 179–202.

Condran, G. A., & Crimmins-Gardner, E. (1978). Public health measures and mortality in U.S. cities in the late nineteenth century. *Human Ecology*, *6*(1), 27–54. https://doi.org/10.1007/BF00888565.

Crimmins, E. M. (1981). The changing pattern of American mortality decline, 1940–77, and its implications for the future. *Population and Development Review*, 7(2), 229–254. https://doi.org/10.2307/1972622.

Currie, J., & Schwandt, H. (2016). Inequality in mortality decreased among the young while increasing for older adults, 1990–2010. *Science*, *352*(6286), 708–712. https://doi.org/10.1126/science.aaf1437.

Cutler, D., Deaton, A., & Lleras-Muney, A. (2006). The determinants of mortality. *Journal of Economic Perspectives, 20*(3), 97–120. https://doi.org/10.1257/jep.20.3.97.

Cutler, D., & Miller, G. (2005). The role of public health improvements in health advances: The twentieth-century United States. *Demography, 42*(1), 1–22. https://doi.org/10.1353/dem.2005.0002.

Daley, J. (2019, January 2). Was the world's oldest person ever actually her 99-year-old daughter? *Smithsonian Magazine*. www.smithsonianmag.com/smart-news/study-questions-age-worlds-oldest-woman-180971153/.

Denney, J. T., Rogers, R. G., Hummer, R. A., & Pampel, F. C. (2010). Education inequality in mortality: The age and gender specific mediating effects of cigarette smoking. *Social Science Research, 39*(4), 662–673. https://doi.org/10.1016/j.ssresearch.2010.02.007.

Dimick, J., Ruhter, J., Sarrazin, M.V., & Birkmeyer, J. D. (2013). Black patients more likely than whites to undergo surgery at low-quality hospitals in segregated regions. *Health Affairs, 32*(6), 1046–1053. https://doi.org/10.1377/hlthaff.2011.1365.

Douglas, M. R., Manion, C. A., Hall-Harper, V. D., Terronez, K. M., Love, C. A., & Chan, A. (2015). Case studies from community coalitions: Advancing local tobacco control policy in a preemptive state. *American Journal of Preventive Medicine, 48*(1), S29–S35. https://doi.org/10.1016/j.amepre.2014.09.020.

Dupre, M. E. (2007). Educational differences in age-related patterns of disease: Reconsidering the cumulative disadvantage and age-as-leveler hypotheses. *Journal of Health and Social Behavior, 48*(1), 1–15. https://doi.org/10.1177/002214650704800101.

Dupre, M. E. (2008). Educational differences in health risks and illness over the life course: A test of cumulative disadvantage theory. *Social Science Research, 37*(4), 1253–1266. https://doi.org/10.1016/j.ssresearch.2008.05.007.

Easterlin, R. A. (1999). How beneficent is the market? A look at the modern history of mortality. *European Review of Economic History, 3*(3), 257–294. https://doi.org/10.1017/S1361491699000131.

Easterlin, R. A. (2000). The worldwide standard of living since 1800. *Journal of Economic Perspectives, 14*(1), 7–26. https://doi.org/10.1257/jep.14.1.7.

Egen, O., Beatty, K., Blackley, D. J., Brown, K., & Wykoff, R. (2016). Health and social conditions of the poorest versus wealthiest counties in the United States. *American Journal of Public Health, 107*(1), 130–135. https://doi.org/10.2105/AJPH.2016.303515.

Elo, I. T. (2009). *Social class differentials in health and mortality: Patterns and explanations in comparative perspective* (SSRN Scholarly Paper ID 1603405). Social Science Research Network. https://papers.ssrn.com/abstract=1603405.

Engelman, M., Canudas-Romo, V., & Agree, E. M. (2010). The implications of increased survivorship for mortality variation in aging populations. *Population and Development Review, 36*(3), 511–539. https://doi.org/10.1111/j.1728-4457.2010.00344.x.

Everett, B. G., Rogers, R. G., Hummer, R. A., & Krueger, P. M. (2011). Trends in educational attainment by race/ethnicity, nativity, and sex in the United States, 1989–2005. *Ethnic and Racial Studies, 34*(9), 1543–1566. https://doi.org/10.1080/01419870.2010.543139.

Fallin, A., & Glantz, S. A. (2015). Tobacco-control policies in tobacco-growing states: Where tobacco was king. *The Milbank Quarterly, 93*(2), 319–358. https://doi.org/10.1111/1468-0009.12124.

Fields, B. E., Bell, J. F., Moyce, S., & Bigbee, J. L. (2015). The impact of insurance instability on health service utilization: Does non-metropolitan residence make a difference? *The Journal of Rural Health, 31*(1), 27–34. https://doi.org/10.1111/jrh.12077.

Fields, B. E., Bigbee, J. L., & Bell, J. F. (2016). Associations of provider-to-population ratios and population health by county-level rurality. *The Journal of Rural Health*, *32*(3), 235–244. https://doi.org/10.1111/jrh.12143.

Frenk, J., & Gómez-Dantés, O. (2017). False dichotomies in global health: The need for integrative thinking. *The Lancet*, *389*(10069), 667–670. https://doi.org/10.1016/S0140-6736(16)30181-7.

Fuller-Rowell, T. E., Curtis, D. S., Doan, S. N., & Coe, C. L. (2015). Racial disparities in the health benefits of educational attainment: A study of inflammatory trajectories among African American and white adults. *Psychosomatic Medicine*, 77(1), 33. https://doi.org/10.1097/PSY.0000000000000128.

Gavrilova, N. S., & Gavrilov, L. A. (2019). Are we approaching a biological limit to human longevity? *The Journals of Gerontology. Series A, Biological Sciences and Medical Sciences*. https://doi.org/10.1093/gerona/glz164.

Gillum, R. F., Mehari, A., Curry, B., & Obisesan, T. O. (2012). Racial and geographic variation in coronary heart disease mortality trends. *BMC Public Health*, *12*, 410. https://doi.org/10.1186/1471-2458-12-410.

Glymour, M. M., Avendaño, M., & Berkman, L. F. (2007). Is the 'stroke belt' worn from childhood? Risk of first stroke and state of residence in childhood and adulthood. *Stroke*, *38*(9), 2415–2421. https://doi.org/10.1161/STROKEAHA.107.482059.

Gómez, J. E., Johnson, B. A., Selva, M., & Sallis, J. F. (2004). Violent crime and outdoor physical activity among inner-city youth. *Preventive Medicine*, *39*(5), 876–881. https://doi.org/10.1016/j.ypmed.2004.03.019.

Gorman, D. M., Speer, P. W., Gruenewald, P. J., & Labouvie, E. W. (2001). Spatial dynamics of alcohol availability, neighborhood structure and violent crime. *Journal of Studies on Alcohol*, *62*(5), 628–636. https://doi.org/10.15288/jsa.2001.62.628.

Granados, J. A. T. (2005). Increasing mortality during the expansions of the US economy, 1900–1996. *International Journal of Epidemiology*, *34*(6), 1194–1202. https://doi.org/10.1093/ije/dyi141.

Gutierrez, K. S., & LePrevost, C. E. (2016). Climate justice in rural southeastern United States: A review of climate change impacts and effects on human health. *International Journal of Environmental Research and Public Health*, *13*(2), 189. https://doi.org/10.3390/ijerph13020189.

Hayward, M. D., & Gorman, B. K. (2004). The long arm of childhood: The influence of early-life social conditions on men's mortality. *Demography*, *41*(1), 87–107. https://doi.org/10.1353/dem.2004.0005.

Hayward, M. D., Hummer, R. A., & Sasson, I. (2015). Trends and group differences in the association between educational attainment and U.S. adult mortality: Implications for understanding education's causal influence. *Social Science & Medicine*, *127*, 8–18. https://doi.org/10.1016/j.socscimed.2014.11.024.

Heckman, J. J. (2006). Skill formation and the economics of investing in disadvantaged children. *Science*, *312*(5782), 1900–1902. https://doi.org/10.1126/science.1128898.

Herd, P. (2010). Education and health in late-life among high school graduates: Cognitive versus psychological aspects of human capital. *Journal of Health and Social Behavior*, *51*(4), 478–496. https://doi.org/10.1177/0022146510386796.

Hobbes, T. (1886). *Leviathan; or, the matter, form and power of a commonwealth, ecclesiastical and civil*. George Routledge and Sons.

Holt, J. B., Zhang, X., Presley-Cantrell, L., & Croft, J. B. (2011). Geographic disparities in chronic obstructive pulmonary disease (COPD) hospitalization among Medicare beneficiaries in the United States. *International Journal of Chronic Obstructive Pulmonary Disease, 6*, 321–328. https://doi.org/10.2147/COPD.S19945.

Houle, J. N. (2014). Disparities in debt: Parents' socioeconomic resources and young adult student loan debt. *Sociology of Education, 87*(1), 53–69. https://doi.org/10.1177/0038040713512213.

Hout, M. (2012). Social and economic returns to college education in the United States. *Annual Review of Sociology, 38*(1), 379–400. https://doi.org/10.1146/annurev.soc.012809.102503.

Howell, J., & Elliott, J. R. (2019). Damages done: The longitudinal impacts of natural hazards on wealth inequality in the United States. *Social Problems, 66*(3), 448–467. https://doi.org/10.1093/socpro/spy016.

Hummer, R. A., & Hernandez, E. M. (2013). The effect of educational attainment on adult mortality in the United States. *Population Bulletin, 68*(1), 1–16.

Iqbal, N. (2011, October 19). The secret of the world's oldest marathon runner. *The Guardian*. www.theguardian.com/uk/2011/oct/19/secret-worlds-oldest-marathon-runner-100.

James, W., & Cossman, J. S. (2017). Long-term trends in Black and white mortality in the rural United States: Evidence of a race-specific rural mortality penalty. *The Journal of Rural Health, 33*(1), 21–31. https://doi.org/10.1111/jrh.12181.

James, W. L. (2014). All rural places are not created equal: Revisiting the rural mortality penalty in the United States. *American Journal of Public Health, 104*(11), 2122–2129. https://doi.org/10.2105/AJPH.2014.301989.

Johansson, S. R. (1994). Food for thought: Rhetoric and reality in modern mortality history. *Historical Methods: A Journal of Quantitative and Interdisciplinary History, 27*(3), 101–125. https://doi.org/10.1080/01615440.1994.10594227.

Johansson, S. R., & Mosk, C. (1987). Exposure, resistance and life expectancy: Disease and death during the economic development of Japan, 1900–1960. *Population Studies, 41*(2), 207–235.

Jones, D. E., Greenberg, M., & Crowley, M. (2015). Early social-emotional functioning and public health: The relationship between kindergarten social competence and future wellness. *American Journal of Public Health, 105*(11), 2283–2290. https://doi.org/10.2105/AJPH.2015.302630.

Jones, D. S., Podolsky, S. H., & Greene, J. A. (2012). The burden of disease and the changing task of medicine. *New England Journal of Medicine, 366*(25), 2333–2338. https://doi.org/10.1056/NEJMp1113569.

Khazan, O. (2017, December 21). A shocking decline in American life expectancy. *The Atlantic*. www.theatlantic.com/health/archive/2017/12/life-expectancy/548981/.

Khera, R., Vaughan-Sarrazin, M., Rosenthal, G. E., & Girotra, S. (2015). Racial disparities in outcomes after cardiac surgery: The role of hospital quality. *Current Cardiology Reports, 17*(5), 29. https://doi.org/10.1007/s11886-015-0587-7.

Kitagawa, E. M., & Hauser, P. M. (1973). *Differential mortality in the United States: A study in socioeconomic epidemiology*. Harvard University Press.

Knowles, J. H. (1977). The responsibility of the individual. *Daedalus, 106*(1), 57–80.

Kulkarni, S. C., Levin-Rector, A., Ezzati, M., & Murray, C. J. (2011). Falling behind: Life expectancy in U.S. counties from 2000 to 2007 in an international context. *Population Health Metrics, 9*, 16. https://doi.org/10.1186/1478-7954-9-16.

Lee, K.-S. (2007). Infant mortality decline in the late 19th and early 20th centuries: The role of market milk. *Perspectives in Biology and Medicine, 50*(4), 585–602. https://doi.org/10.1353/pbm.2007.0051.

Ma, J., Ward, E. M., Siegel, R. L., & Jemal, A. (2015). Temporal trends in mortality in the United States, 1969–2013. *Journal of the American Medical Association, 314*(16), 1731–1739. https://doi.org/10.1001/jama.2015.12319.

Ma, J., Xu, J., Anderson, R. N., & Jemal, A. (2012). Widening educational disparities in premature death rates in twenty six states in the United States, 1993–2007. *PLOS ONE*, 7(7), e41560. https://doi.org/10.1371/journal.pone.0041560.

Masters, R. K., Hummer, R. A., & Powers, D. A. (2012). Educational differences in U.S. adult mortality: A cohort perspective. *American Sociological Review*, 77(4), 548–572. https://doi.org/10.1177/0003122412451019.

Masters, R. K., Link, B. G., & Phelan, J. C. (2015). Trends in education gradients of 'preventable' mortality: A test of fundamental cause theory. *Social Science & Medicine, 127*, 19–28. https://doi.org/10.1016/j.socscimed.2014.10.023.

Mathers, C. D., Stevens, G. A., Boerma, T., White, R. A., & Tobias, M. I. (2015). Causes of international increases in older age life expectancy. *The Lancet, 385*(9967), 540–548. https://doi.org/10.1016/S0140-6736(14)60569-9.

McAlpin, M. B. (1983). Famines, epidemics, and population growth: The case of India. *The Journal of Interdisciplinary History, 14*(2), 351–366. https://doi.org/10.2307/203709.

McKenzie, K., Fingerhut, L., Walker, S., Harrison, A., & Harrison, J. E. (2012). Classifying external causes of injury: History, current approaches, and future directions. *Epidemiologic Reviews, 34*(1), 4–16. https://doi.org/10.1093/epirev/mxr014.

McKeown, T. (1976). *The modern rise of population*. Edward Arnold.

McKeown, T. (1979). *The role of medicine: Dream, mirage, or nemesis?* Princeton University Press.

McKeown, T., & Brown, R. G. (1955). Medical evidence related to English population changes in the eighteenth century. *Population Studies, 9*(2), 119–141. https://doi.org/10.1080/00324728.1955.10404688.

Meyer, J. (2012). *Centenarians: 2010* (No. C2010SR-03). United States Census Bureau. www.census.gov/library/publications/2012/dec/c2010sr-03.html.

Miech, R., Pampel, F., Kim, J., & Rogers, R. G. (2011). The enduring association between education and mortality: The role of widening and narrowing disparities. *American Sociological Review, 76*(6), 913–934. https://doi.org/10.1177/0003122411411276.

Mirowsky, J., & Ross, C. E. (2003). *Education, social status, and health*. Transaction Publishers.

Mokdad, A. H., Dwyer-Lindgren, L., Fitzmaurice, C., Stubbs, R. W., Bertozzi-Villa, A., Morozoff, C., Charara, R., Allen, C., Naghavi, M., & Murray, C. J. L. (2017). Trends and patterns of disparities in cancer mortality among U.S. counties, 1980–2014. *Journal of the American Medical Association, 317*(4), 388–406. https://doi.org/10.1001/jama.2016.20324.

Montez, J. K. (2017). Deregulation, devolution, and state preemption laws' impact on U.S. mortality trends. *American Journal of Public Health, 107*(11), 1749–1750. http://dx.doi.org/10.2105/AJPH.2017.304080.

Montez, J. K., & Barnes, K. (2016). The benefits of educational attainment for U.S. adult mortality: Are they contingent on the broader environment? *Population Research and Policy Review, 35*(1), 73–100. https://doi.org/10.1007/s11113-015-9377-6.

Montez, J. K., & Hayward, M. D. (2014). Cumulative childhood adversity, educational attainment, and active life expectancy among U.S. adults. *Demography, 51*(2), 413–435. https://doi.org/10.1007/s13524-013-0261-x.

Montez, J. K., Hayward, M. D., & Wolf, D. A. (2017). Do U.S. states' socioeconomic and policy contexts shape adult disability? *Social Science & Medicine, 178*, 115–126. https://doi.org/10.1016/j.socscimed.2017.02.012.

Montez, J. K., Hummer, R. A., & Hayward, M. D. (2012). Educational attainment and adult mortality in the United States: A systematic analysis of functional form. *Demography*, *49*(1), 315–336. https://doi.org/10.1007/s13524-011-0082-8.

Montez, J. K., Hummer, R. A., Hayward, M. D., Woo, H., & Rogers, R. G. (2011). Trends in the educational gradient of U.S. adult mortality from 1986 through 2006 by race, gender, and age group. *Research on Aging*, *33*(2), 145–171. https://doi.org/10.1177/0164027510392388.

Mosher, J. F., & Treffers, R. D. (2013). State pre-emption, local control, and alcohol retail outlet density regulation. *American Journal of Preventive Medicine*, *44*(4), 399–405. https://doi.org/10.1016/j.amepre.2012.11.029.

Murphy, S. L., Xu, J., Kochanek, K., & Arias, E. (2018). *Mortality in the United States, 2017* (NCHS Data Brief No. 328). National Center for Health Statistics. www.cdc.gov/nchs/products/databriefs/db328.htm.

Nandi, A., Glymour, M. M., & Subramanian, S. V. (2014). Association among socioeconomic status, health behaviors, and all-cause mortality in the United States. *Epidemiology*, *25*(2), 170. https://doi.org/10.1097/EDE.0000000000000038.

National Center for Education Statistics. (2019). *Digest of education statistics, 2017* (No. 2018–070). U.S. Department of Education. https://nces.ed.gov/fastfacts/display.asp?id=76.

National Center for Health Statistics. (2017). *Health, United States, 2016*. www.cdc.gov/nchs/data/hus/hus16.pdf#020.

National Center for Health Statistics. (2018). *Deaths and mortality*. www.cdc.gov/nchs/fastats/deaths.htm.

Nixon, L., Mejia, P., Cheyne, A., Wilking, C., Dorfman, L., & Daynard, R. (2015). "We're part of the solution": Evolution of the food and beverage industry's framing of obesity concerns between 2000 and 2012. *American Journal of Public Health*, *105*(11), 2228–2236. https://doi.org/10.2105/AJPH.2015.302819.

Nutbeam, D. (2008). The evolving concept of health literacy. *Social Science & Medicine*, *67*(12), 2072–2078. https://doi.org/10.1016/j.socscimed.2008.09.050.

Office of Minority Health. (2019). *Profile: Black/African Americans*. U.S. Department of Health and Human Services. www.minorityhealth.hhs.gov/omh/browse.aspx?lvl=3&lvlid=61.

Olshansky, S. J., Antonucci, T., Berkman, L., Binstock, R. H., Boersch-Supan, A., Cacioppo, J. T., Carnes, B. A., Carstensen, L. L., Fried, L. P., Goldman, D. P., Jackson, J., Kohli, M., Rother, J., Zheng, Y., & Rowe, J. (2012). Differences in life expectancy due to race and educational differences are widening, and many may not catch up. *Health Affairs*, *31*(8), 1803–1813. https://doi.org/10.1377/hlthaff.2011.0746.

Omran, A. R. (1971). The epidemiologic transition: A theory of the epidemiology of population change. *The Milbank Quarterly*, *49*(4), 509–538. https://doi.org/10.1111/j.1468-0009.2005.00398.x.

Omran, A. R. (1988). The epidemiologic transition theory revisited thirty years later. *World Health Statistics Quarterly*, *51*(2–4), 99–119.

Oster, E. (2018). *Behavioral feedback: Do individual choices influence scientific results?* [National Bureau of Economic Research Working Paper]. National Bureau of Economic Research. https://doi.org/10.3386/w25225.

Pampel, F., Legleye, S., Goffette, C., Piontek, D., Kraus, L., & Khlat, M. (2015). Cohort changes in educational disparities in smoking: France, Germany and the United States. *Social Science & Medicine*, *127*, 41–50. https://doi.org/10.1016/j.socscimed.2014.06.033.

Pertschuk, M., Hobart, R., Paloma, M., Larkin, M. A., & Balbach, E. D. (2013). Grassroots movement building and preemption in the campaign for residential fire sprinklers. *American Journal of Public Health, 103*(10), 1780–1787. https://doi.org/10.2105/AJPH.2013.301317.

Pertschuk, M., Pomeranz, J. L., Aoki, J. R., Larkin, M. A., & Paloma, M. (2013). Assessing the impact of federal and state preemption in public health: A framework for decision makers. *Journal of Public Health Management and Practice, 19*(3), 213. https://doi.org/10.1097/PHH.0b013e3182582a57.

Peters, D. J., Monnat, S. M., Hochstetler, A. L., & Berg, M. T. (2019). The opioid hydra: Understanding overdose mortality epidemics and syndemics across the rural-urban continuum. *Rural Sociology*. https://doi.org/10.1111/ruso.12307.

Pew Research Center. (2019). *5 facts about student loans*. www.pewresearch.org/fact-tank/2019/08/13/facts-about-student-loans/.

Pickett, K. E., & Wilkinson, R. G. (2015). Income inequality and health: A causal review. *Social Science & Medicine, 128*, 316–326. https://doi.org/10.1016/j.socscimed.2014.12.031.

Polednak, A. P. (2011). Trends in mortality from COPD in selected U.S. states differing in tobacco control efforts. *COPD: Journal of Chronic Obstructive Pulmonary Disease*, 7(1), 63–69. https://doi.org/10.3109/15412550903499514.

Pomeranz, J. L., & Pertschuk, M. (2017). State preemption: A significant and quiet threat to public health in the United States. *American Journal of Public Health, 107*(6), 900–902. https://doi.org/10.2105/AJPH.2017.303756.

Preston, S. H. (1975). The changing relation between mortality and level of economic development. *Population Studies, 29*(2), 231–248. https://doi.org/10.2307/2173509.

Preston, S. H., & Elo, I. T. (1995). Are educational differentials in adult mortality increasing in the United States? *Journal of Aging and Health*, 7(4), 476–496. https://doi.org/10.1177/089826439500700402.

Robert Wood Johnson Foundation. (2015). *Birth place and life expectancy: A look at American cities*. www.rwjf.org/en/library/articles-and-news/2015/09/city-maps.html.

Rogers, R. G., Everett, B. G., Zajacova, A., & Hummer, R. A. (2010). Educational degrees and adult mortality risk in the United States. *Biodemography and Social Biology, 56*(1), 80–99. https://doi.org/10.1080/19485561003727372.

Roser, M. (2019). *Life expectancy*. https://ourworldindata.org/life-expectancy.

Roush, S. W., Murphy, T. V., & Group, and the V.-P. D. T. W. (2007). Historical comparisons of morbidity and mortality for vaccine-preventable diseases in the United States. *Journal of the American Medical Association, 298*(18), 2155–2163. https://doi.org/10.1001/jama.298.18.2155.

Santacreu, A. M., & Zhu, H. (2017). *How does U.S. income inequality compare worldwide?* Federal Reserve Bank of St. Louis. www.stlouisfed.org/on-the-economy/2017/october/how-us-income-inequality-compare-worldwide.

Sasson, I. (2016). Trends in life expectancy and lifespan variation by educational attainment: United States, 1990–2010. *Demography, 53*(2), 269–293. https://doi.org/10.1007/s13524-015-0453-7.

Schafer, M. H., Wilkinson, L. R., & Ferraro, K. F. (2013). Childhood (mis)fortune, educational attainment, and adult health: Contingent benefits of a college degree? *Social Forces, 91*(3), 1007–1034. https://doi.org/10.1093/sf/sos192.

Scutchfield, F. D., & Keck, C. W. (2017). Deaths of despair: Why? What to do? *American Journal of Public Health, 107*(10), 1564–1565. http://dx.doi.org.proxy.bc.edu/10.2105/AJPH.2017.303992.

Semega, J., Kollar, M., Creamer, J., & Mohanty, A. (2019). *Income and poverty in the United States: 2018* [P60–266]. United States Census Bureau. www.census.gov/library/publications/2019/demo/p60-266.html.

Singh, G. K., Kogan, M. D., & Slifkin, R. T. (2017). Widening disparities in infant mortality and life expectancy between Appalachia and the rest of the United States, 1990–2013. *Health Affairs, 36*(8), 1423–1432. https://doi.org/10.1377/hlthaff.2016.1571.

Singh, G. K., & Siahpush, M. (2014). Widening rural–urban disparities in life expectancy, U.S., 1969–2009. *American Journal of Preventive Medicine, 46*(2), e19–e29. https://doi.org/10.1016/j.amepre.2013.10.017.

Smits, J., & Monden, C. (2009). Length of life inequality around the globe. *Social Science & Medicine, 68*(6), 1114–1123. https://doi.org/10.1016/j.socscimed.2008.12.034.

Sommers, B. D., Baicker, K., & Epstein, A. M. (2012). Mortality and access to care among adults after state Medicaid expansions. *New England Journal of Medicine, 367*(11), 1025–1034. https://doi.org/10.1056/NEJMsa1202099.

Spencer, C. S., Gaskin, D. J., & Roberts, E. T. (2013). The quality of care delivered to patients within the same hospital varies by insurance type. *Health Affairs, 32*(10), 1731–1739. https://doi.org/10.1377/hlthaff.2012.1400.

Stuart, A. L., Mudhasakul, S., & Sriwatanapongse, W. (2009). The social distribution of neighborhood-scale air pollution and monitoring protection. *Journal of the Air & Waste Management Association, 59*(5), 591–602. https://doi.org/10.3155/1047-3289.59.5.591.

Szreter, S. (1988). The importance of social intervention in Britain's mortality decline c.1850–1914: A re-interpretation of the role of public health. *Social History of Medicine, 1*(1), 1–38. https://doi.org/10.1093/shm/1.1.1.

Szreter, S. (2002). Rethinking McKeown: The relationship between public health and social change. *American Journal of Public Health, 92*(5), 722–725. https://doi.org/10.2105/AJPH.92.5.722.

Thornton, R. L. J., Glover, C. M., Cené, C. W., Glik, D. C., Henderson, J. A., & Williams, D. R. (2016). Evaluating strategies for reducing health disparities by addressing the social determinants of health. *Health Affairs, 35*(8), 1416–1423. https://doi.org/10.1377/hlthaff.2015.1357.

Tomes, N. (1990). The private side of public health: Sanitary science, domestic hygiene, and the germ theory, 1870–1900. *Bulletin of the History of Medicine, 64*(4), 509–539.

Uhlenberg, P. (1980). Death and the family. *Journal of Family History, 5*(3), 313–320. https://doi.org/10.1177/036319908000500304.

U.S. Department of Health & Human Services. (2018). *Global statistics*. www.hiv.gov/hiv-basics/overview/data-and-trends/global-statistics.

Virginia Commonwealth University Center on Society and Health. (2016). *Mapping life expectancy*. https://societyhealth.vcu.edu/work/the-projects/mapping-life-expectancy.html.

Walsemann, K. M., Hummer, R. A., & Hayward, M. D. (2018). Heterogeneity in educational pathways and the health behavior of U.S. young adults. *Population Research and Policy Review*, 1–24. https://doi.org/10.1007/s11113-018-9463-7.

Warren, J. R. (2016). Does growing childhood socioeconomic inequality mean future inequality in adult health? *The ANNALS of the American Academy of Political and Social Science, 663*(1), 292–330. https://doi.org/10.1177/0002716215596981.

Western, B., Bloome, D., & Percheski, C. (2008). Inequality among American families with children, 1975 to 2005. *American Sociological Review, 73*(6), 903–920. https://doi.org/10.1177/000312240807300602.

Woolf, S. H., & Braveman, P. (2011). Where health disparities begin: The role of social and economic determinants – and why current policies may make matters worse. *Health Affairs*, *30*(10), 1852–1859. https://doi.org/10.1377/hlthaff.2011.0685.

World Bank. (2019). *Prevalence of HIV*. https://data.worldbank.org/indicator/SH.DYN.AIDS.ZS?year_low_desc=true.

World Health Organization. (2016). *Life expectancy at birth, 2000–2016: Both sexes*. http://gamapserver.who.int/gho/interactive_charts/mbd/life_expectancy/atlas.html.

Yamashita, T., & Kunkel, S. R. (2010). The association between heart disease mortality and geographic access to hospitals: County level comparisons in Ohio, USA. *Social Science & Medicine*, *70*(8), 1211–1218. https://doi.org/10.1016/j.socscimed.2009.12.028.

Zajacova, A. (2012). Health in working-aged Americans: Adults with high school equivalency diploma are similar to dropouts, not high school graduates. *American Journal of Public Health*, *102*(S2), S284–S290. https://doi.org/10.2105/AJPH.2011.300524.

Zajacova, A., & Everett, B. G. (2014). The nonequivalent health of high school equivalents. *Social Science Quarterly*, *95*(1), 221–238. https://doi.org/10.1111/ssqu.12039.

Zenk, S. N., Powell, L. M., Isgor, Z., Rimkus, L., Barker, D. C., & Chaloupka, F. J. (2015). Prepared food availability in U.S. food stores: A national study. *American Journal of Preventive Medicine*, *49*(4), 553–562. https://doi.org/10.1016/j.amepre.2015.02.025.

Zheng, H., & George, L. K. (2018). Does medical expansion improve population health? *Journal of Health and Social Behavior*, *59*(1), 113–132. https://doi.org/10.1177/0022146518754534.

PART I

Private Troubles

3

LIFE'S FINAL WEEKS

If death is now predictable, then what can we predict about the quality of the last weeks of life? In this chapter, I describe the quality of the typical, predictable death in the U.S. today, and explain the cultural and economic reasons for this situation. I go on to contrast this common experience with both lay and scholarly ideas about how deaths should ideally happen. I assess the strengths and weaknesses of the hospice movement and the Medicare hospice benefit, mechanisms for providing more comfortable, peaceful predictable deaths. I conclude by examining the large racial and ethnic disparities in who is and is not able to receive goal-concordant end-of-life care in the U.S. today.

Typical Death

In the 1990s and early 2000s, a series of major reports drew attention to the sorry state of dying patients in the United States. A National Academies report highlighted the high frequency of shortness of breath, pain, anxiety, cognitive impairment – ranging from confusion to complete non-responsiveness – and immobility in the last weeks of life (Institute of Medicine, 1997). Then, the Study to Understand Prognoses and Preferences for Outcomes and Risks of Treatments (SUPPORT) created still more controversy. In its first phase, this study examined patients with advanced illnesses who received care at five teaching hospitals over a two-year period. It documented a number of alarming results, including that 47% of patients had doctors who did not know whether and in what circumstances the patient wanted standard treatments such as cardiopulmonary resuscitation (CPR; Connors, 1995). SUPPORT included a second phase, a two-year randomized controlled trial in the same hospitals. Nearly 5,000 patients participated in phase 2. Each patient was assigned a specially trained nurse whose job was to facilitate communication among patients, their families, and the various health care professionals who were treating the patient. Additionally, physicians received continuing education about prognosis and about the efficacy of common medical interventions for dying persons (Murphy et al., 2000).

There were five targeted outcomes, including physician knowledge of the patient's treatment preferences, and the study results showed no improvement on *any* of the five outcomes. A flurry of research attempted to identify methodological flaws in the study, but no flaw could account for the null results (Lynn, DeVries, et al., 2000). The study left many health care professionals, policymakers, and medical researchers reckoning with their assumptions about delivering good care at the end of life (Lynn, Arkes, et al., 2000), yet despite this wake-up call, there are few signs that conditions for dying people have improved in the interim. Symptoms such as pain, anxiety or depression, confusion, and shortness of breath are all as common or more common than they were at the turn of the century (Singer et al., 2015; Teno et al., 2015).

These symptoms occur despite, or perhaps because of, high rates of hospitalization and intensive use of life-sustaining treatments. Most people would prefer to avoid hospitals, yet about one-fifth of U.S. deaths occur in hospitals (Dartmouth Institute for Health Policy and Clinical Practice, 2019).[1] Moreover, two-thirds of people are hospitalized at some time in their last six months of life, often more than once, for an average of eight days (Dartmouth Institute for Health Policy and Clinical Practice, 2019). A related concern is the average of 3.1 transitions among hospital, home, and various types of long-term care facilities in the last months of life (Teno et al., 2013). Fourteen percent of patients experience a transition in the last 3 days of life. Such transitions are disruptive to the patient and family, and destabilizing to the patient's condition when they produce discontinuities in care across facilities.

With regard to life sustaining treatment, the average patient is taking an average of 11 prescription medications at the time of death (McNeil et al., 2016). Other common treatments include mechanical ventilation, CPR, artificial nutrition and hydration, and hemodialysis. More than half of critically ill people report that they would rather be dead than live with these interventions (Rubin et al., 2016). Nonetheless, health care professionals often do not obtain the patient's informed consent before beginning these therapies (Teno, Mitchell, et al., 2011).

Despite their widespread use, intensive interventions produce marginal returns to both short-term and long-term survival (Barnato et al., 2010). Half of people who spend any time receiving life-sustaining treatments will die within 6 months (Detsky et al., 2017). *Non-beneficial* treatment is the most value-neutral term used to refer to interventions that do not produce improvements in quality of life, in health status, or in the likelihood of improving enough to leave the hospital (Cardona-Morrell et al., 2016). Other researchers condemn the use of such treatment more explicitly, calling it "futile" (Schneiderman, 2011, p. 123), "low value" (de Vries et al., 2016, p. 1) and "potentially inappropriate" (Kon et al., 2016, p. 1769).

The extent of non-beneficial treatment is extremely difficult to assess, because even two medical professionals examining the same case may disagree on whether care produced meaningful improvements (Neville et al., 2015). However, in one sample of New York City physicians, 91% said that they had given treatment that they considered to be futile or potentially inappropriate (Lambden et al., 2019). Given that patient autonomy is a key value in modern medicine, another potential standard for whether care is beneficial is whether the care meets the patient's goals (Brudney, 2009). A recent estimate is that approximately 13% of deaths include care that is discordant with patients' goals, with a higher rate – 30% – among patients with dementia (Ernecoff et al., 2018; Khandelwal et al., 2017).

Why Is Care for the Typical Death So Intensive?

In theory, the changes of the epidemiological transition opened opportunities for the predictable death to be comfortable, peaceful, and even meaningful. People should have the agency to enact their care preferences and end their lives on their own terms. Why, then, does the typical death involve a high-symptom burden and care that may be non-beneficial? The theory of medicalization sheds some light on this problem. Medicalization occurs when "a medical frame or definition has been applied to understand or manage a problem" such as death (Conrad, 1992). In the early 1980s, cultural historian Aries (1982) traced the medicalization of death over 1,000 years of Western society. He suggests that in the past, death was a misfortune, but was routine and even familiar. As the Enlightenment progressed in Europe, death became subject to rationalization. Then people began to consider death to be unnatural, and wanted experts who could predict, monitor, treat, delay, and otherwise control it.

Thus, the job of "brokering" death, or making it acceptable to patients and their survivors, has fallen to health care providers (Timmermans, 2005, p. 993). Ideas about the most appropriate practices to broker death can change in relatively short periods of time. For example, in 1960, 90% of physicians thought that a cancer patient should not be told his or her diagnosis, but by 1980, 97% of physicians thought that a cancer patient should be told (Novack et al., 1979). Ironically, the goal of these two opposite practices was the same: Health care professionals are loathe to do anything that they fear might cause the patient or family to lose hope. As many studies show, the will to live has prognostic value (Carmel et al., 2007; Karppinen et al., 2012).

However, how to maintain hope is largely still a matter of individual health care professionals' clinical judgement. Doctors are extremely reluctant to pronounce how much time a patient has left (Christakis, 1999). Almost all doctors will explain that a condition is terminal, but less than half volunteer a time frame unless the patient requests one (Daugherty & Hlubocky, 2008). In part, doctors withhold a prognosis because many diseases continue to have a large degree of uncertainty. For example, half of congestive heart failure patients die within five years of diagnosis, while the other half survive more than five years (Mozaffarian et al., 2016). However, while a majority of doctors say they believe that patients should have all available information about their prognosis, many admit that they have nevertheless withheld information from a patient because they were concerned that he or she would lose hope (Hancock et al., 2007). Yet about 70% of patients say that they want to know their prognosis, and on average, patients experience less, rather than more, emotional distress when their physicians are forthcoming about a terminal prognosis (Enzinger et al., 2015; Fried et al., 2006; Yun et al., 2010).

In addition to maintaining hope, another responsibility of physicians who are brokering death is to exhaust all medical options. In her book *Ordinary medicine*, Sharon Kaufman describes the four steps by which extraordinary medical interventions become ordinary or normative (Kaufman, 2015). First, biomedical researchers make discoveries, which are tested in human clinical trials and approved by accrediting bodies (in the U.S., the Food and Drug Administration). Next, insurers decide which innovations they will and will not reimburse. These decisions in effect form the toolkit of possible treatments that health care professionals can draw upon, because patients can rarely pay for treatment without the aid of insurance. Thus treatments that insurers cover become norms of care, and doctors and patients feel an almost moral imperative to try at least some, if not all, of the tools in the toolkit to preserve the patient's life (Shim et al., 2008).

In her earlier book, *… And a time to die*, Kaufman explained how successive tests of interventions in the toolkit produce "the revolving door" (Kaufman, 2005, p. 131). Repeatedly, chronically ill patients encounter life-threatening situations, and then modern medicine saves them, again and again. Other scholars have called this cycle *clinical momentum* because it becomes difficult for health care providers, families, and patients to stop to evaluate the usefulness of specific interventions in the context of a patient's goals, preferences, and likely prognosis (Kruser et al., 2016). Lynn and colleagues (Lynn, Arkes, et al., 2000) came to posit that one reason the SUPPORT trial failed is that it rested on the assumption that stakeholders would recognize major decision-points in a patient's trajectory, when in practice these points passed by as routine instances for medical intervention.

Eventually, the revolving door stops when medicine fails. The occasion of death comes as something of a surprise to the people immersed in this situation, even when the patient was extremely ill (Russ & Kaufman, 2005). Health care professionals are often unprepared as well, and thus sometimes regard a patient who succumbs to terminal illness as a sign of professional failure (Kaufman, 2010). Education on death and dying in U.S. medical schools is improving (Dickinson, 2006); however, many medical students never care for a dying patient during their training (Anderson et al., 2008). Later, as physicians, they have not learned how to cope with their own sense of loss when a patient dies under their care, nor to broker the situation for others (Kearney et al., 2009).

Both hesitancy about communicating prognostic information and the phenomenon of clinical momentum result in decision-making that makes sense at the time, but appears unfortunate in retrospect. For example, non-beneficial care is often the result of these processes, such as when a physician feels uncertain about a prognosis and fears that the family might file a malpractice lawsuit if he or she leaves treatments untried (Jox et al., 2012; Palda et al., 2005). A longstanding call in bioethics is that a change in medical culture towards an "ethic of care" and away from an "ethic of cure" may reduce these problems (Šarić et al., 2017; Schneiderman et al., 1994, p. 110). That is, if comfort becomes a more important goal than survival, then care practices should follow.

However, the mindsets of health care professionals, families, and patients are not the only forces promoting intensive treatment regardless of benefit. Health care systems, which are structured as businesses in the U.S., face financial pressures. In 2013, for example, 55% of hospitals failed to earn a profit (Bai & Anderson, 2016). Consequently, there is a push for hospitals to offer more profitable services and fewer unprofitable services (Bekes et al., 2004; Horwitz, 2005). Profitable services include critical care medicine such as cardiac intensive care as well as advanced imaging procedures such as MRI and PET scans (Horwitz & Nichols, 2009) Unprofitable services include less technology-dependent services such as psychiatric care and geriatric day care programs (Horwitz & Nichols, 2009). Against such market forces, simply promoting an ethic of care will likely be insufficient to improve the typical death.

Good Death

Most health care providers, patients, and their families generally agree on the characteristics of the death they would prefer, and they are quite different from the characteristics of the typical death. People want pain and symptom management, socioemotional and, for many, religious or spiritual support, dignity and quality of life (Meier et al., 2016; Steinhauser et al., 2000). Aries (1982) termed this a *good* death. People have agreed on the central characteristics of a good death since at least the Middle Ages (Granda-Cameron & Houldin, 2012), but there is great variation in ideas about the best way to achieve a good death.

Some of this variation is due to misinformation: Many people express a desire to receive certain medical interventions because they are unfamiliar with the level of pain and invasiveness involved, the proportion of patients who survive them, and the quality of life of patients who survive them (Shif et al., 2015). For example, about 40% of people believe that three-quarters of people who undergo CPR survive and recover sufficiently to leave the hospital, when in fact only a fifth actually survive to discharge (Donohoe et al., 2006; Morrison et al., 2013). People tend to acquire their information from sources such as television medical dramas that are designed to entertain, not to educate (e.g., Brodie et al., 2001; Harris & Willoughby, 2009). Comparatively, physicians have more accurate knowledge about how these interventions can and cannot help achieve a good death, and request their own treatment accordingly. Physicians are less likely than non-physicians to die in a hospital, less likely to have surgery in the last 6 months of life, and less likely to spend time in the intensive care unit in their last 6 months of life (Weissman et al., 2016).

However, some of the variation in ideas about good death is due to true differences in preference. Some people see the greatest dignity in resisting their disease, for example, whereas others find dignity in quiet acceptance of their own mortality (Clow, 2001). Thus there is a danger in stating that any objective measure, such as having an ICU admission in the last week of life, represents a death that was not good. Instead, researchers think about good death in terms of goal concordance, or whether patients receive care that enables them to experience whatever is personally most important (Sanders et al., 2017). For example, a patient may wish to live long enough to say goodbye to a relative traveling from far away, and may be willing to endure ICU treatment to increase the chances of realizing that goal.

The goals that patients most often list concern the dying process (Meier et al., 2016), such as where they will die, who will and will not be with them, and how they will die (e.g., in sleep). Patients may hold contradictory goals, especially soon after they receive their prognosis, and so a person's goals may evolve with time and with experience with the health care system. For example, although the low proportion of deaths at home is often held up as an example of goal-discordant care, scholars warn that a home death is not the best option for everyone (Pollock, 2015). Patients who are able to die at home have support from health care providers, as well as strong social support from family and friends (Gomes & Higginson, 2006). Without such support, a home death may not be a good death for people who do not have adequate nursing, or for people who are socially isolated. Additionally, a home death can be stressful for survivors, who are often faced with providing what amounts to critical care medicine without the resources of a hospital or the training of a nurse or physician (Moorman & Macdonald, 2013). Although patients do frequently express a wish to die at home in their own beds, they may later decide that other goals outweigh their desire to die at home, and that another type of facility would better help them to attain those goals (MacArtney et al., 2016).

Palliative Care, Hospice, and the Good Death

Despite the current distance between the typical death and the good death, there are models for excellent care for the dying. Palliative care, designed to alleviate both physical and psychosocial symptoms, can occur simultaneously with treatments designed to cure disease or heal injury. For example, a cancer patient can undergo chemotherapy and also have effective pain management. Most professional organizations in medicine recommend that patients receive both palliative care and curative care beginning at diagnosis (Smith et al., 2012). Patients who begin palliative care early in the course of their disease survive longer than people who begin palliative care late in the course of their disease (Bakitas et al., 2015).

Medicare, which insures Americans 65 and older, is the reason that the words *palliative care* are nearly synonymous with death and dying in the collective conscious. Medicare pays a hospice benefit for palliative care for persons aged 65 and older, provided that a doctor has issued a prognosis of six months or less, and that the patient has agreed to forgo subsequent curative treatment (Centers for Medicare and Medicaid Services, 2019). Thus, hospice is palliative care designed specifically for people who are dying. In 2016, 48% of decedents were receiving the Medicare hospice benefit at the time of death (National Hospice and Palliative Care Organization, 2017).

Since 1982, the Medicare hospice benefit has provided palliative care for patients who are in the terminal stages of their illness and have stopped seeking a cure; however, the term *hospice* has a history much longer than that of the Medicare benefit. The word originally referred to a shelter for long-distance travelers in medieval Europe. Modern hospice is a philosophy of care for people with life-limiting disease, and some characterize it as a social movement to change medicine (Siebold, 1992). The movement is generally traced to Cecily Saunders, a British nurse and eventual physician who, until her death in 2005, wrote and spoke extensively about care for dying and bereaved people. Dr. Saunders envisioned hospice as supportive care for what she called "total pain," or the emotional, psychological, social, and spiritual distress that people experience in addition to physical distress (Saunders, 2006, p. 87).

Easing total pain includes several elements that are distinct from those of traditional medicine. One is that dying persons should not be isolated in spaces away from people who are not dying. Often this means care at home, but effective social integration can occur in institutions such as hospitals or nursing homes as well. A second element is that the family, rather than the patient, is considered to be the unit of care. Everyone in the family may experience total pain surrounding the death. A third element is that an interdisciplinary team coordinates care, including not only doctors and nurses, but also psychiatrists, social workers, clergy, and even volunteers. Thus therapies may be non-medical or in the realm of alternative medicine, including massage, music therapy, and other means of symptom reduction (Gutgsell et al., 2013). Beyond these three elements, there is great variation in the delivery of the hospice benefit in terms of the settings in which people receive care, the professionals involved in the care team, and the specific services that are available (Carlson et al., 2007).

The effectiveness of hospice is difficult to evaluate because of this variability in delivery, the feasibility and bioethics involved in conducting research with dying and bereaved people, and the selectivity of who enrolls in hospice. That is, not only are some physicians, such as oncologists who work in not-for-profit systems, more likely to refer their patients to hospice than others, but also hospice patients' individual characteristics, such as race/ethnicity and diagnosis, differ from those of other decedents (Lepore et al., 2011; Obermeyer et al., 2015) Nonetheless, scholars have developed innovative models for studying hospice (Casarett et al., 2012; Wohleber et al., 2012). I review the highest quality research here.

The efficacy of hospice is generally evaluated by major illness category. For example, scholars review the evidence for hospice care for patients with dementia (Teno, Gozalo, et al., 2011), or for hospice care for patients with kidney disease (Murray et al., 2006). The literature takes this form because common symptoms, types of treatment, and intensity of care differ dramatically across major illness categories. For example, shortness of breath is a very distressing symptom that is more common in chronic lower respiratory diseases than it is of most types of cancer, and so lower respiratory patients experience higher rates of mechanical ventilation in standard care than cancer patients do. In addition to these physiological differences across disease type, specialists' levels of familiarity and comfort with death and dying, knowledge about symptom palliation, and expectations about the possible returns to treatment vary across disease type. Cancer and dementia patients have a good probability of dying outside of the ICU or hospital and of receiving goal-concordant care, while lower respiratory disease patients and end-stage renal disease patients often receive more intensive, hospital-based intervention (Wachterman et al., 2016; Wong et al., 2012).

Nevertheless, across illness categories, hospice patients differ from non-hospice patients on a number of important dimensions. First, thanks to palliative care, hospice patients receive more comprehensive symptom control than dying patients who are not in hospice care (Higginson & Evans, 2010). Consequently, they are better able to meet their personal goals, and report better quality life in their final days as well as greater satisfaction with the end-of-life care they have received (Bakitas et al., 2009; Gade et al., 2008). Finally, care in hospice involves markedly less medical intervention than standard care: People who enroll in hospice are less likely to die in the hospital and less likely to experience hospitalizations and other transitions in their last months than people who receive standard care (Kelley et al., 2013).

Other important benefits of hospice concern outcomes for family and other loved ones. Hospice programs provide practical support to care providers to the dying, as well as emotional support, opportunities for communication, and preparation for bereavement. Some services continue after the death (Cherlin et al., 2007). Bereaved family members of hospice patients report greater satisfaction with the quality of the care the decedent received than do family members of patients who received standard care (Teno, Gozalo, et al., 2011). Hospice also affects care-workers' coping and quality of life, and after the death, their experience of grief (Northouse et al., 2010). Following a death, family members whose loved one spent a short duration (three days or less) in hospice were more likely to experience major depressive disorder than family members who had more contact with hospice (Kris et al., 2006). Hospice may even affect the mortality of bereaved people. Usually, bereaved spouses have an increased risk of dying themselves within the first year or two of widowhood. Hospice care may eliminate this risk (Christakis & Iwashyna, 2003).

Hospice care has been a bright spot in efforts to improve quality of care at the end of life: The proportion of people who were receiving the Medicare hospice benefit when they die doubled, to 42%, over the ten-year period 2000–2010, and rose to 48% by 2016 (National Hospice and Palliative Care Organization, 2017; Teno et al., 2013). This expansion was not a major driver of increases in health care costs (Brooks et al., 2014; Gozalo et al., 2015). In 2016 alone, 4,382 hospices provided a median of 24 days of care to 1.43 million people under the Medicare hospice benefit. The Medicare hospice benefit certainly permits patients to access hospice who otherwise would be unable to afford such services.

Nevertheless, hospice faces two major challenges. First, to qualify for the benefit, patients must have a prognosis of six or fewer months of life. Such a prognosis is relatively straightforward for diseases that have predictable trajectories, such as most types of cancer, but much less straightforward for other conditions, such as congestive heart failure. Because doctors are typically overly optimistic in their prognoses, patients who could benefit from hospice services are not eligible for them because their prognoses are longer than six months (Glare et al., 2003). Hospice patients who do survive beyond six months can continue to receive services, paid for by Medicare, so long as they continue to decline. Patients whose condition stabilizes are disqualified and lose their benefits (Luth et al., 2020). In fact, 21% of hospice patients are discharged alive from the program (Russell et al., 2017).

However, the cause of most live discharges is not disqualification, but rather acute hospitalization (Russell et al., 2017). The second major challenge to hospice is that patients must entirely forgo curative, life-saving care in order to receive the hospice benefit. Distressed care workers observe disturbing symptoms and call 911, often not understanding that a hospitalization ends hospice eligibility (Ankuda et al., 2017; Phongtankuel et al., 2016).

Moreover, patients, families, and health care providers who do understand this provision are often reluctant to commit to forgo curative care and enroll in hospice. Thus, over a quarter of hospice patients die after receiving services for a week or less (National Hospice and Palliative Care Organization, 2017). In fact, patients who never enter hospice at all receive less medical intervention in the last six months of life than do brief-stay hospice patients, who receive high-intensity curative care until their deaths are imminent (Aldridge & Bradley, 2017). A short hospice stay may help make the moment of death itself physically comfortable, but the hospice model works best when it has time to address the psychosocial and spiritual elements of total pain.

Racial/Ethnic Disparities in the Good Death

Race/ethnicity is a pervasive and troubling fundamental cause of both mortality and the quality of death, with an especially large differential between Black and

White Americans. Indeed, it is difficult to identify areas of health care that are not shaped by racial and ethnic disparities. From conception throughout the life course, Americans of color are sicker and more likely to die than Whites Americans (National Center for Health Statistics, 2016). They are at greater risk of almost all chronic and infectious diseases, and their age at disease onset is younger than it is among Whites. Persons of color are more likely than Whites to have multiple diseases simultaneously, which means that they have medical crises more often as well (Soto et al., 2013). Persons of color develop more severe and complex cases of illness than Whites because they are less likely to have access to preventive care or early treatment (Soto et al., 2013). Both at the hospital and in the community, persons of color receive poorer quality health care and less of it, with longer wait times than Whites. They are also more likely to experience complications such as sepsis following medical procedures (Mayr et al., 2010).

When they are dying, Americans of color continue to receive poorer quality health care, yet they begin to receive *more* intensive medical intervention than White people do. Due to greater exposure to cigarette smoke and other environmental toxins, people of color are more likely than Whites to have respiratory diseases and other illnesses that are generally treated intensively at the end of life (Celedón et al., 2014). Persons of color are more likely than Whites to: die in the intensive care unit and in the hospital; be admitted to the hospital in their last year of life; and receive life-sustaining interventions in their last year of life (Barnato et al., 2007; Tschirhart et al., 2014). Persons of color are less likely than Whites to: be satisfied with the quality of their end-of-life care (Lee et al., 2016); report adequate symptom control and effective communication with their health care providers (Johnson, 2013); and use hospice services (LoPresti et al., 2016).

The cause of all of these disparities is racism, working in interrelated ways at all levels of society (Phelan & Link, 2015). Here, I address three of those ways: residential segregation, low-socioeconomic status, and patient concerns about discrimination. First, residential segregation by race and ethnicity continues to be pervasive in the United States (Massey, 2015) and persists in long-term care settings (Davis et al., 2014). There is evidence that reducing residential segregation improves health among persons of color (Kershaw et al., 2017; LaVeist et al., 2011). Residential segregation has at least two consequences for health: (a) persons of color live and work in communities that have high exposure to health risks, and (b) persons of color live and work in communities with low-quality health care services. Communities in which persons of color are segregated tend to be located in places that have a host of direct risks to health, such as air pollution (Jones et al., 2014). Additionally, persons of color are more likely than Whites to get curative treatment in settings that have quality and intensity of care problems for *all* of their patients (Barnato et al., 2017). These settings frequently have high patient loads, unmet staffing needs, and insufficient funding. People of all races and ethnicities who are treated in these hospitals have poorer short- and long-term outcomes than people who are treated at higher-quality institutions

(Khera et al., 2015). However, hospice care shows pervasive racial disparities regardless of residential segregation, with Black patients more likely than White patients to be discharged alive from the same hospice (Rizzuto & Aldridge, 2018).

Second, as a group, persons of color in the United States have less educational attainment, lower incomes, less wealth, and lower job prestige than White Americans (Chetty et al., 2019). Socioeconomic status (SES) is a strong predictor of all-cause mortality for people of all racial and ethnic backgrounds (Signorello et al., 2014). Because the U.S. does not have public health insurance for younger adults, SES affects access to insurance until one is old enough to qualify for Medicare. Even within Medicare, people who have more money can buy higher-quality care (Joynt et al., 2017). High-socioeconomic status also permits individuals to purchase resources for health that are outside of the healthcare system, such as a residence in a healthy, racially integrated neighborhood. Finally, high-socioeconomic status is an indicator of access to knowledge and information about diseases, their symptoms, and their treatments, as well as how to advocate for oneself in the health care system successfully (Tieu et al., 2017). For example, low income and educational attainment are barriers to hospice availability, accessibility, and acceptability (Lewis et al., 2011)

Third, patients of color and their families are well aware of the racial/ethnic disparities in almost every aspect of health and health care, and they are also well aware of both historical and contemporary cases of explicit racism and exploitation of black and brown bodies in medicine. Therefore, persons of color anticipate that they will receive goal discordant care when they are dying (LoPresti et al., 2016). Black Americans are more likely than Whites to want aggressive medical intervention, because they do not trust health care providers to give them all possible options (Johnson et al., 2008). Black families who do use hospice rate even hospices with a greater proportion of Black patients, which might be expected to be more culturally sensitive, more poorly than they rate hospices that primarily serve White patients (Rhodes et al., 2012). Hispanic Americans tend to want palliative care, but often experience communication difficulties with their health care providers, especially if English is not a first language (Kelley et al., 2010). For many Hispanic migrants, the U.S. healthcare system's emphasis on individual autonomy over shared family decision-making is confusing and off-putting (Yennurajalingam et al., 2013).

Summary

This chapter has described the typical predictable death in the U.S. today. It involves distressing physical symptoms that prevent patients from achieving their final goals despite extensive, sometimes non-beneficial, medical intervention. Hospice is an alternative model of care for dying persons and their families that accounts for suffering that is psychosocial as well as suffering that is physical. Approximately half of people who die in the U.S. are receiving hospice services when they die; however, the most common pattern is for people to receive extensive medical intervention until just a few days before death, whereupon they enter hospice. Further, persons of color are less likely than White Americans to receive hospice services, because of persistent racism in the health care system. Therefore, hospice use is not as widespread as it may need to be to improve death quality in the U.S. Changes to Medicare that allow people to couple hospice and curative care may help this problem.

Note

1. Other common places that people die include at home and in a long-term care facility such as a nursing home (Aldridge & Bradley, 2017).

References

Aldridge, M. D., & Bradley, E. H. (2017). Epidemiology and patterns of care at the end of life: Rising complexity, shifts in care patterns and sites of death. *Health Affairs, 36*(7), 1175–1183. https://doi.org/10.1377/hlthaff.2017.0182.

Anderson, W. G., Williams, J. E., Bost, J. E., & Barnard, D. (2008). Exposure to death is associated with positive attitudes and higher knowledge about end-of-life care in graduating medical students. *Journal of Palliative Medicine, 11*(9), 1227–1233. https://doi.org/10.1089/jpm.2008.0058.

Ankuda, C. K., Fonger, E., & O'Neil, T. (2017). Electing full code in hospice: Patient characteristics and live discharge rates. *Journal of Palliative Medicine, 21*(3), 297–301. https://doi.org/10.1089/jpm.2017.0276.

Aries, P. (1982). *The hour of our death*. Penguin Random House.

Bai, G., & Anderson, G. F. (2016). A more detailed understanding of factors associated with hospital profitability. *Health Affairs, 35*(5), 889–897. https://doi.org/10.1377/hlthaff.2015.1193.

Bakitas, M., Lyons, K. D., Hegel, M. T., Balan, S., Brokaw, F. C., Seville, J., Hull, J. G., Li, Z., Tosteson, T. D., Byock, I. R., & Ahles, T. A. (2009). Effects of a palliative care intervention on clinical outcomes in patients with advanced cancer: The project ENABLE II randomized controlled trial. *Journal of the American Medical Association, 302*(7), 741–749. https://doi.org/10.1001/jama.2009.1198.

Bakitas, M. A., Tosteson, T. D., Li, Z., Lyons, K. D., Hull, J. G., Li, Z., Dionne-Odom, J. N., Frost, J., Dragnev, K. H., Hegel, M. T., Azuero, A., & Ahles, T. A. (2015). Early versus delayed initiation of concurrent palliative oncology care: Patient outcomes in the ENABLE III randomized controlled trial. *Journal of Clinical Oncology, 33*(13), 1438–1445. https://doi.org/10.1200/JCO.2014.58.6362.

Barnato, A. E., Chang, C.-C. H., Farrell, M. H., Lave, J. R., Roberts, M. S., & Angus, D. C. (2010). Is survival better at hospitals with higher "end-of-life" treatment intensity? *Medical Care, 48*(2), 125–132. https://doi.org/10.1097/MLR.0b013e3181c161e4.

Barnato, A. E., Chang, C.-C. H., Lave, J. R., & Angus, D. C. (2017). The paradox of end-of-life hospital treatment intensity among black patients: A retrospective cohort study. *Journal of Palliative Medicine, 21*(1), 69–77. https://doi.org/10.1089/jpm.2016.0557.

Barnato, A. E., Chang, C.-C. H., Saynina, O., & Garber, A. M. (2007). Influence of race on inpatient treatment intensity at the end of life. *Journal of General Internal Medicine, 22*(3), 338–345. https://doi.org/10.1007/s11606-006-0088-x.

Bekes, C. E., Dellinger, R. P., Brooks, D., Edmondson, R., Olivia, C. T., & Parrillo, J. E. (2004). Critical care medicine as a distinct product line with substantial financial profitability: The role of business planning. *Critical Care Medicine, 32*(5), 1207–1214. https://doi.org/10.1097/01.CCM.0000126152.33719.DB.

Brodie, M., Foehr, U., Rideout, V., Baer, N., Miller, C., Flournoy, R., & Altman, D. (2001). Communicating health information through the entertainment media. *Health Affairs, 20*(1), 192–199. https://doi.org/10.1377/hlthaff.20.1.192.

Brooks, G. A., Li, L., Uno, H., Hassett, M. J., Landon, B. E., & Schrag, D. (2014). Acute hospital care is the chief driver of regional spending variation in Medicare patients with advanced cancer. *Health Affairs, 33*(10), 1793–1800. https://doi.org/10.1377/hlthaff.2014.0280.

Brudney, D. (2009). Beyond autonomy and best interests. *Hastings Center Report, 39*(2), 31–37. https://doi.org/10.1353/hcr.0.0113.

Cardona-Morrell, M., Kim, J. C. H., Turner, R. M., Anstey, M., Mitchell, I. A., & Hillman, K. (2016). Non-beneficial treatments in hospital at the end of life: A systematic review on extent of the problem. *International Journal for Quality in Health Care, 28*(4), 456–469. https://doi.org/10.1093/intqhc/mzw060.

Carlson, M. D. A., Morrison, R. S., Holford, T. R., & Bradley, E. H. (2007). Hospice care: What services do patients and their families receive? *Health Services Research, 42*(4), 1672–1690. https://doi.org/10.1111/j.1475-6773.2006.00685.x.

Carmel, S., Baron-Epel, O., & Shemy, G. (2007). The will-to-live and survival at old age: Gender differences. *Social Science & Medicine, 65*(3), 518–523. https://doi.org/10.1016/j.socscimed.2007.03.034.

Casarett, D. J., Harrold, J., Oldanie, B., Prince-Paul, M., & Teno, J. (2012). Advancing the science of hospice care: Coalition of hospices organized to investigate comparative effectiveness. *Current Opinion in Supportive and Palliative Care, 6*(4), 459. https://doi.org/10.1097/SPC.0b013e32835a66b7.

Celedón, J. C., Roman, J., Schraufnagel, D. E., Thomas, A., & Samet, J. (2014). Respiratory health equality in the United States. The American Thoracic Society perspective. *Annals of the American Thoracic Society, 11*(4), 473–479. https://doi.org/10.1513/AnnalsATS.201402-059PS.

Centers for Medicare and Medicaid Services. (2019). *Medicare hospice benefits* (No. 02154). www.medicare.gov/Publications/.

Cherlin, E. J., Barry, C. L., Prigerson, H. G., Green, D. S., Johnson-Hurzeler, R., Kasl, S.V., & Bradley, E. H. (2007). Bereavement services for family caregivers: How often used, why, and why not. *Journal of Palliative Medicine, 10*(1), 148–158. https://doi.org/10.1089/jpm.2006.0108.

Chetty, R., Hendren, N., Jones, M. R., & Porter, S. R. (2019). *Race and economic opportunity in the United States: An intergenerational perspective* (No. 24441). National Bureau of Economic Research. www.nber.org/papers/w24441.

Christakis, N. A. (1999). *Death Foretold*. www.press.uchicago.edu/ucp/books/book/chicago/D/bo3641373.html.

Christakis, N. A., & Iwashyna, T. J. (2003). The health impact of health care on families: A matched cohort study of hospice use by decedents and mortality outcomes in surviving, widowed spouses. *Social Science & Medicine, 57*(3), 465–475. https://doi.org/10.1016/S0277-9536(02)00370-2.

Clow, B. (2001). Who's afraid of Susan Sontag? Or, the myths and metaphors of cancer reconsidered. *Social History of Medicine, 14*(2), 293–312. https://doi.org/10.1093/shm/14.2.293.

Connors, A. F. (1995). A controlled trial to improve care for seriously ill hospitalized patients: The study to understand prognoses and preferences for outcomes and risks of treatments (SUPPORT). *Journal of the American Medical Association, 274*(20), 1591. https://doi.org/10.1001/jama.1995.03530200027032.

Conrad, P. (1992). Medicalization and social control. *Annual Review of Sociology, 18*, 209–232.

Dartmouth Institute for Health Policy and Clinical Practice. (2019). *Dartmouth atlas of health care*. www.dartmouthatlas.org/data/table.aspx?ind=15.

Daugherty, C. K., & Hlubocky, F. J. (2008). What are terminally ill cancer patients told about their expected deaths? A study of cancer physicians' self-reports of prognosis disclosure. *Journal of Clinical Oncology, 26*(36), 5988–5993. https://doi.org/10.1200/JCO.2008.17.2221.

Davis, J. A., Weech-Maldonado, R., Lapane, K. L., & Laberge, A. (2014). Contextual determinants of U.S. nursing home racial/ethnic diversity. *Social Science & Medicine, 104*, 142–147. https://doi.org/10.1016/j.socscimed.2013.12.009.

de Vries, E. F., Struijs, J. N., Heijink, R., Hendrikx, R. J. P., & Baan, C. A. (2016). Are low-value care measures up to the task? A systematic review of the literature. *BMC Health Services Research, 16*, 405. https://doi.org/10.1186/s12913-016-1656-3.

Detsky, M. E., Harhay, M. O., Bayard, D. F., Delman, A. M., Buehler, A. E., Kent, S. A., Ciuffetelli, I. V., Cooney, E., Gabler, N. B., Ratcliffe, S. J., Mikkelsen, M. E., & Halpern, S. D. (2017). Six-month morbidity and mortality among intensive care unit patients receiving life-sustaining therapy. A prospective cohort study. *Annals of the American Thoracic Society, 14*(10), 1562–1570. https://doi.org/10.1513/AnnalsATS.201611-875OC.

Dickinson, G. E. (2006). Teaching end-of-life issues in U.S. medical schools: 1975 to 2005. *American Journal of Hospice and Palliative Medicine, 23*(3), 197–204. https://doi.org/10.1177/1049909106289066.

Donohoe, R. T., Haefeli, K., & Moore, F. (2006). Public perceptions and experiences of myocardial infarction, cardiac arrest and CPR in London. *Resuscitation, 71*(1), 70–79. https://doi.org/10.1016/j.resuscitation.2006.03.003.

Enzinger, A. C., Zhang, B., Schrag, D., & Prigerson, H. G. (2015). Outcomes of prognostic disclosure: Associations with prognostic understanding, distress, and relationship with physician among patients with advanced cancer. *Journal of Clinical Oncology, 33*(32), 3809–3816. https://doi.org/10.1200/JCO.2015.61.9239.

Ernecoff, N. C., Zimmerman, S., Mitchell, S. L., Song, M.-K., Lin, F.-C., Wessell, K. L., & Hanson, L. C. (2018). Concordance between goals of care and treatment decisions for persons with dementia. *Journal of Palliative Medicine, 21*(10), 1442–1447. https://doi.org/10.1089/jpm.2018.0103.

Fried, T. R., Bradley, E. H., & O'Leary, J. (2006). Changes in prognostic awareness among seriously ill older persons and their caregivers. *Journal of Palliative Medicine, 9*(1), 61–69. https://doi.org/10.1089/jpm.2006.9.61.

Gade, G., Venohr, I., Conner, D., McGrady, K., Beane, J., Richardson, R. H., Williams, M. P., Liberson, M., Blum, M., & Penna, R. D. (2008). Impact of an inpatient palliative care team: A randomized controlled trial. *Journal of Palliative Medicine, 11*(2), 180–190. https://doi.org/10.1089/jpm.2007.0055.

Glare, P., Virik, K., Jones, M., Hudson, M., Eychmuller, S., Simes, J., & Christakis, N. (2003). A systematic review of physicians' survival predictions in terminally ill cancer patients. *British Medical Journal, 327*(7408), 195. https://doi.org/10.1136/bmj.327.7408.195.

Gomes, B., & Higginson, I. J. (2006). Factors influencing death at home in terminally ill patients with cancer: Systematic review. *British Medical Journal, 332*(7540), 515–521. https://doi.org/10.1136/bmj.38740.614954.55.

Gozalo, P., Plotzke, M., Mor, V., Miller, S. C., & Teno, J. M. (2015). Changes in Medicare costs with the growth of hospice care in nursing homes. *New England Journal of Medicine, 372*(19), 1823–1831. https://doi.org/10.1056/NEJMsa1408705.

Granda-Cameron, C., & Houldin, A. (2012). Concept analysis of good death in terminally ill patients. *American Journal of Hospice and Palliative Medicine, 29*(8), 632–639. https://doi.org/10.1177/1049909111434976.

Gutgsell, K. J., Schluchter, M., Margevicius, S., DeGolia, P. A., McLaughlin, B., Harris, M., Mecklenburg, J., & Wiencek, C. (2013). Music therapy reduces pain in palliative care patients: A randomized controlled trial. *Journal of Pain and Symptom Management, 45*(5), 822–831. https://doi.org/10.1016/j.jpainsymman.2012.05.008.

Hancock, K., Clayton, J. M., Parker, S. M., der, S. W., Butow, P. N., Carrick, S., Currow, D., Ghersi, D., Glare, P., Hagerty, R., & Tattersall, M. H. (2007). Truth-telling in discussing prognosis in advanced life-limiting illnesses: A systematic review. *Palliative Medicine, 21*(6), 507–517. https://doi.org/10.1177/0269216307080823.

Harris, D., & Willoughby, H. (2009). Resuscitation on television: Realistic or ridiculous? A quantitative observational analysis of the portrayal of cardiopulmonary resuscitation in television medical drama. *Resuscitation, 80*(11), 1275–1279. https://doi.org/10.1016/j.resuscitation.2009.07.008.

Higginson, I. J., & Evans, C. J. (2010). What is the evidence that palliative care teams improve outcomes for cancer patients and their families? *The Cancer Journal, 16*(5), 423. https://doi.org/10.1097/PPO.0b013e3181f684e5.

Horwitz, J. R. (2005). Making profits and providing care: Comparing nonprofit, for-profit, and government hospitals. *Health Affairs, 24*(3), 790–801. https://doi.org/10.1377/hlthaff.24.3.790.

Horwitz, J. R., & Nichols, A. (2009). Hospital ownership and medical services: Market mix, spillover effects, and nonprofit objectives. *Journal of Health Economics, 28*(5), 924–937. https://doi.org/10.1016/j.jhealeco.2009.06.008.

Institute of Medicine. (1997). *Approaching death: Improving care at the end of life*. National Academies Press.

Johnson, K. S. (2013). Racial and ethnic disparities in palliative care. *Journal of Palliative Medicine, 16*(11), 1329–1334. https://doi.org/10.1089/jpm.2013.9468.

Johnson, K. S., Kuchibhatla, M., & Tulsky, J. A. (2008). What explains racial differences in the use of advance directives and attitudes toward hospice care? *Journal of the American Geriatrics Society, 56*(10), 1953–1958. https://doi.org/10.1111/j.1532-5415.2008.01919.x.

Jones, M. R., Diez-Roux, A. V., Hajat, A., Kershaw, K. N., O'Neill, M. S., Guallar, E., Post, W. S., Kaufman, J. D., & Navas-Acien, A. (2014). Race/ethnicity, residential segregation, and exposure to ambient air pollution: The multi-ethnic study of atherosclerosis (MESA). *American Journal of Public Health, 104*(11), 2130–2137. https://doi.org/10.2105/AJPH.2014.302135.

Jox, R. J., Schaider, A., Marckmann, G., & Borasio, G. D. (2012). Medical futility at the end of life: The perspectives of intensive care and palliative care clinicians. *Journal of Medical Ethics*, medethics-2011-100479. https://doi.org/10.1136/medethics-2011-100479.

Joynt, K. E., De Lew, N., Sheingold, S. H., Conway, P. H., Goodrich, K., & Epstein, A. M. (2017). Should Medicare value-based purchasing take social risk into account? *New England Journal of Medicine, 376*(6), 510–513. https://doi.org/10.1056/NEJMp1616278.

Karppinen, H., Laakkonen, M.-L., Strandberg, T. E., Tilvis, R. S., & Pitkälä, K. H. (2012). Will-to-live and survival in a 10-year follow-up among older people. *Age and Ageing, 41*(6), 789–794. https://doi.org/10.1093/ageing/afs082.

Kaufman, S. R. (2005). *And a time to die*. University of Chicago Press.

Kaufman, S. R. (2010). Time, clinic technologies, and the making of reflexive longevity: The cultural work of time left in an ageing society. *Sociology of Health & Illness, 32*(2), 225–237. https://doi.org/10.1111/j.1467-9566.2009.01200.x.

Kaufman, S. R. (2015). *Ordinary medicine*. Duke University Press.

Kearney, M. K., Weininger, R. B., Vachon, M. L. S., Harrison, R. L., & Mount, B. M. (2009). Self-care of physicians caring for patients at the end of life: "Being connected … a key to my survival." *Journal of the American Medical Association, 301*(11), 1155–1164. https://doi.org/10.1001/jama.2009.352.

Kelley, A. S., Deb, P., Du, Q., Aldridge Carlson, M. D., & Morrison, R. S. (2013). Hospice enrollment saves money for Medicare and improves care quality across a number of different lengths-of-stay. *Health Affairs, 32*(3), 552–561. https://doi.org/10.1377/hlthaff.2012.0851.

Kelley, A. S., Wenger, N. S., & Sarkisian, C. A. (2010). Opiniones: End-of-life care preferences and planning of older Latinos. *Journal of the American Geriatrics Society, 58*(6), 1109–1116. https://doi.org/10.1111/j.1532-5415.2010.02853.x.

Kershaw, K. N., Robinson, W. R., Gordon-Larsen, P., Hicken, M. T., Goff, D. C., Carnethon, M. R., Kiefe, C. I., Sidney, S., & Roux, A. V. D. (2017). Association of changes in neighborhood-level racial residential segregation with changes in blood pressure among Black adults: The CARDIA study. *Journal of the American Medical Association Internal Medicine, 177*(7), 996–1002. https://doi.org/10.1001/jamainternmed.2017.1226.

Khandelwal, N., Curtis, J. R., Freedman, V. A., Kasper, J. D., Gozalo, P., Engelberg, R. A., & Teno, J. M. (2017). How often is end-of-life care in the United States inconsistent with patients' goals of care? *Journal of Palliative Medicine, 20*(12), 1400–1404. https://doi.org/10.1089/jpm.2017.0065.

Khera, R., Vaughan-Sarrazin, M., Rosenthal, G. E., & Girotra, S. (2015). Racial disparities in outcomes after cardiac surgery: The role of hospital quality. *Current Cardiology Reports, 17*(5), 29. https://doi.org/10.1007/s11886-015-0587-7.

Kon, A. A., Shepard, E. K., Sederstrom, N. O., Swoboda, S. M., Marshall, M. F., Birriel, B., & Rincon, F. (2016). Defining futile and potentially inappropriate interventions: A policy statement from the Society of Critical Care Medicine Ethics Committee. *Critical Care Medicine, 44*(9), 1769. https://doi.org/10.1097/CCM.0000000000001965.

Kris, A. E., Cherlin, E. J., Prigerson, H., Carlson, M. D. A., Johnson-Hurzeler, R., Kasl, S.V., & Bradley, E. H. (2006). Length of hospice enrollment and subsequent depression in family caregivers: 13-month follow-up study. *The American Journal of Geriatric Psychiatry, 14*(3), 264–269. https://doi.org/10.1097/01.JGP.0000194642.86116.ce.

Kruser, J. M., Cox, C. E., & Schwarze, M. L. (2016). Clinical momentum in the intensive care unit. A latent contributor to unwanted care. *Annals of the American Thoracic Society, 14*(3), 426–431. https://doi.org/10.1513/AnnalsATS.201611-931OI.

Lambden, J. P., Chamberlin, P., Kozlov, E., Lief, L., Berlin, D. A., Pelissier, L. A., Yushuvayev, E., Pan, C. X., & Prigerson, H. G. (2019). Association of perceived futile or potentially inappropriate care with burnout and thoughts of quitting among health-care providers. *American Journal of Hospice and Palliative Medicine®, 36*(3), 200–206. https://doi.org/10.1177/1049909118792517.

LaVeist, T., Pollack, K., Thorpe, R., Fesahazion, R., & Gaskin, D. (2011). Place, not race: Disparities dissipate in southwest Baltimore when Blacks and Whites live under similar conditions. *Health Affairs, 30*(10), 1880–1887. https://doi.org/10.1377/hlthaff.2011.0640.

Lee, J. J., Long, A. C., Curtis, J. R., & Engelberg, R. A. (2016). The influence of race/ethnicity and education on family ratings of the quality of dying in the ICU. *Journal of Pain and Symptom Management, 51*(1), 9–16. https://doi.org/10.1016/j.jpainsymman.2015.08.008.

Lepore, M. J., Miller, S. C., & Gozalo, P. (2011). Hospice use among urban Black and White U.S. nursing home decedents in 2006. *The Gerontologist, 51*(2), 251–260. https://doi.org/10.1093/geront/gnq093.

Lewis, J. M., DiGiacomo, M., Currow, D. C., & Davidson, P. M. (2011). Dying in the margins: Understanding palliative care and socioeconomic deprivation in the developed world. *Journal of Pain and Symptom Management, 42*(1), 105–118. https://doi.org/10.1016/j.jpainsymman.2010.10.265.

LoPresti, M. A., Dement, F., & Gold, H. T. (2016). End-of-life care for people with cancer from ethnic minority groups: A systematic review. *American Journal of Hospice and Palliative Medicine, 33*(3), 291–305. https://doi.org/10.1177/1049909114565658.

Luth, E. A., Russell, D. J., Brody, A. A., Dignam, R., Czaja, S. J., Ryvicker, M., Bowles, K. H., & Prigerson, H. G. (2020). Race, ethnicity, and other risks for live discharge among hospice patients with dementia. *Journal of the American Geriatrics Society. 68*(3), 551–558. https://doi.org/10.1111/jgs.16242.

Lynn, J., Arkes, H. R., Stevens, M., Cohn, F., Koenig, B., Fox, E., Dawson, N. V., Phillips, R. S., Hamel, M. B., & Tsevat, J. (2000). Rethinking fundamental assumptions: SUPPORT'S implications for future reform. *Journal of the American Geriatrics Society, 48*(S1), S214–S221. https://doi.org/10.1111/j.1532-5415.2000.tb03135.x.

Lynn, J., DeVries, K. O., Arkes, H. R., Stevens, M., Cohn, F., Murphy, P., Covinsky, K. E., Hamel, M. B., Dawson, N. V., & Tsevat, J. (2000). Ineffectiveness of the SUPPORT intervention: Review of explanations. *Journal of the American Geriatrics Society, 48*(S1). https://doi.org/10.1111/j.1532-5415.2000.tb03134.x.

MacArtney, J. I., Broom, A., Kirby, E., Good, P., Wootton, J., & Adams, J. (2016). Locating care at the end of life: Burden, vulnerability, and the practical accomplishment of dying. *Sociology of Health & Illness, 38*(3), 479–492. https://doi.org/10.1111/1467-9566.12375.

Massey, D. S. (2015). The legacy of the 1968 Fair Housing Act. *Sociological Forum, 30*(S1), 571–588. https://doi.org/10.1111/socf.12178.

Mayr, F. B., Yende, S., Linde-Zwirble, W. T., Peck-Palmer, O. M., Barnato, A. E., Weissfeld, L. A., & Angus, D. C. (2010). Infection rate and acute organ dysfunction risk as explanations for racial differences in severe sepsis. *Journal of the American Medical Association, 303*(24), 2495–2503. https://doi.org/10.1001/jama.2010.851.

McNeil, M. J., Kamal, A. H., Kutner, J. S., Ritchie, C. S., & Abernethy, A. P. (2016). The burden of polypharmacy in patients near the end of life. *Journal of Pain and Symptom Management, 51*(2), 178–183.e2. https://doi.org/10.1016/j.jpainsymman.2015.09.003.

Meier, E. A., Gallegos, J. V., Thomas, L. P. M., Depp, C. A., Irwin, S. A., & Jeste, D. V. (2016). Defining a good death (successful dying): Literature review and a call for research and public dialogue. *The American Journal of Geriatric Psychiatry, 24*(4), 261–271. https://doi.org/10.1016/j.jagp.2016.01.135.

Moorman, S. M., & Macdonald, C. (2013). Medically complex home care and caregiver strain. *The Gerontologist, 53*(3), 407–417. https://doi.org/10.1093/geront/gns067.

Morrison, L. J., Neumar, R. W., Zimmerman, J. L., Link, M. S., Newby, L. K., McMullan, P. W., Hoek, T. V., Halverson, C. C., Doering, L., Peberdy, M. A., & Edelson, D. P. (2013). Strategies for improving survival after in-hospital cardiac arrest in the United States. *Circulation, 127*(14), 1538–1563. https://doi.org/10.1161/CIR.0b013e31828b2770.

Mozaffarian, D., J., B. E., Go Alan S., Arnett Donna K., Blaha Michael J., Cushman Mary, Das Sandeep R., de Ferranti Sarah, Després Jean-Pierre, Fullerton Heather J., Howard Virginia J., Huffman Mark D., Isasi Carmen R., Jiménez Monik C., Judd Suzanne E., Kissela Brett M., Lichtman Judith H., Lisabeth Lynda D., Liu Simin, … Turner Melanie B. (2016). Heart disease and stroke statistics – 2016 update. *Circulation, 133*(4), e38–e360. https://doi.org/10.1161/CIR.0000000000000350.

Murphy, P., Kreling, B., Kathryn, E., Stevens, M., Lynn, J., & Dulac, J. (2000). Description of the SUPPORT intervention. *Journal of the American Geriatrics Society, 48*(5 Suppl), S154–161.

Murray, A. M., Arko, C., Chen, S.-C., Gilbertson, D. T., & Moss, A. H. (2006). Use of hospice in the United States dialysis population. *Clinical Journal of the American Society of Nephrology, 1*(6), 1248–1255. https://doi.org/10.2215/CJN.00970306.

National Center for Health Statistics. (2016). *Health, United States, 2015*. www.ncbi.nlm.nih.gov/books/NBK367640/.

National Hospice and Palliative Care Organization. (2017). *Facts and figures: Hospice care in America*. www.nhpco.org/sites/default/files/public/Statistics_Research/2017_Facts_Figures.pdf.

Neville, T. H., Wiley, J. F., Yamamoto, M. C., Flitcraft, M., Anderson, B., Curtis, J. R., & Wenger, N. S. (2015). Concordance of nurses and physicians on whether critical care patients are receiving futile treatment. *American Journal of Critical Care, 24*(5), 403–410. https://doi.org/10.4037/ajcc2015476.

Northouse, L. L., Katapodi, M. C., Song, L., Zhang, L., & Mood, D. W. (2010). Interventions with family caregivers of cancer patients: Meta-analysis of randomized trials. *CA: A Cancer Journal for Clinicians, 60*(5), 317–339. https://doi.org/10.3322/caac.20081.

Novack, D. H., Plumer, R., Smith, R. L., Ochitill, H., Morrow, G. R., & Bennett, J. M. (1979). Changes in physicians' attitudes toward telling the cancer patient. *Journal of the American Medical Association, 241*(9), 897–900. https://doi.org/10.1001/jama.1979.03290350017012.

Obermeyer, Z., Powers, B. W., Makar, M., Keating, N. L., & Cutler, D. M. (2015). Physician characteristics strongly predict patient enrollment in hospice. *Health Affairs, 34*(6), 993–1000. https://doi.org/10.1377/hlthaff.2014.1055.

Palda, V. A., Bowman, K. W., McLean, R. F., & Chapman, M. G. (2005). "Futile" care: Do we provide it? Why? A semistructured, Canada-wide survey of intensive care unit doctors and nurses. *Journal of Critical Care, 20*(3), 207–213. https://doi.org/10.1016/j.jcrc.2005.05.006.

Phelan, J. C., & Link, B. G. (2015). Is racism a fundamental cause of inequalities in health? *Annual Review of Sociology, 41*(1), 311–330. https://doi.org/10.1146/annurev-soc-073014-112305.

Phongtankuel, V., Scherban, B. A., Reid, M. C., Finley, A., Martin, A., Dennis, J., & Adelman, R. D. (2016). Why do home hospice patients return to the hospital? A study of hospice provider perspectives. *Journal of Palliative Medicine, 19*(1), 51–56. https://doi.org/10.1089/jpm.2015.0178.

Pollock, K. (2015). Is home always the best and preferred place of death? *British Medical Journal, 351*. http://dx.doi.org/10.1136/bmj.h4855.

Rhodes, R. L., Xuan, L., & Halm, E. A. (2012). African American bereaved family members' perceptions of hospice quality: Do hospices with high proportions of African Americans do better? *Journal of Palliative Medicine, 15*(10), 1137–1141. https://doi.org/10.1089/jpm.2012.0151.

Rizzuto, J., & Aldridge, M. D. (2018). Racial disparities in hospice outcomes: A race or hospice-level effect? *Journal of the American Geriatrics Society, 66*(2), 407–413. https://doi.org/10.1111/jgs.15228.

Rubin, E. B., Buehler, A. E., & Halpern, S. D. (2016). States worse than death among hospitalized patients with serious illnesses. *Journal of the American Medical Association Internal Medicine, 176*(10), 1557. https://doi.org/10.1001/jamainternmed.2016.4362.

Russ, A. J., & Kaufman, S. R. (2005). Family perceptions of prognosis, silence, and the "suddenness" of death. *Culture, Medicine and Psychiatry, 29*(1), 103–123. https://doi.org/10.1007/s11013-005-4625-6.

Russell, D., Diamond, E. L., Lauder, B., Dignam, R. R., Dowding, D. W., Peng, T. R., Prigerson, H. G., & Bowles, K. H. (2017). Frequency and risk factors for live discharge from hospice. *Journal of the American Geriatrics Society, 65*(8), 1726–1732. https://doi.org/10.1111/jgs.14859.

Sanders, J. J., Curtis, J. R., & Tulsky, J. A. (2017). Achieving goal-concordant care: A conceptual model and approach to measuring serious illness communication and its impact. *Journal of Palliative Medicine, 21*(S2), S-17. https://doi.org/10.1089/jpm.2017.0459.

Šarić, L., Prkić, I., & Jukić, M. (2017). Futile treatment – A review. *Journal of Bioethical Inquiry, 14*(3), 329–337. https://doi.org/10.1007/s11673-017-9793-x.

Saunders, C. (2006). *Selected writings 1958–2004*. Oxford University Press.

Schneiderman, L. J. (2011). Defining medical futility and improving medical care. *Journal of Bioethical Inquiry, 8*(2), 123–131. https://doi.org/10.1007/s11673-011-9293-3.

Schneiderman, L. J., Faber-Langendoen, K., & Jecker, N. S. (1994). Beyond futility to an ethic of care. *The American Journal of Medicine, 96*(2), 110–114. https://doi.org/10.1016/0002-9343(94)90130-9.

Shif, Y., Doshi, P., & Almoosa, K. F. (2015). What CPR means to surrogate decision makers of ICU patients. *Resuscitation, 90*, 73–78. https://doi.org/10.1016/j.resuscitation.2015.02.014.

Shim, J. K., Russ, A. J., & Kaufman, S. R. (2008). Late-life cardiac interventions and the treatment imperative. *PLOS Medicine, 5*(3), e7. https://doi.org/10.1371/journal.pmed.0050007.

Siebold, C. (1992). *The hospice movement: Easing death's pains*. Maxwell Macmillan International.

Signorello, L. B., Cohen, S. S., Williams, D. R., Munro, H. M., Hargreaves, M. K., & Blot, W. J. (2014). Socioeconomic status, race, and mortality: A prospective cohort study. *American Journal of Public Health, 104*(12), e98–e107. https://doi.org/10.2105/AJPH.2014.302156.

Singer, A. E., Meeker, D., Teno, J. M., Lynn, J., Lunney, J. R., & Lorenz, K. A. (2015). Symptom trends in the last year of life from 1998 to 2010: A cohort study. *Annals of Internal Medicine, 162*(3), 175. https://doi.org/10.7326/M13-1609.

Smith, T. J., Temin, S., Alesi, E. R., Abernethy, A. P., Balboni, T. A., Basch, E. M., Ferrell, B. R., Loscalzo, M., Meier, D. E., Paice, J. A., Peppercorn, J. M., Somerfield, M., Stovall, E., & Von Roenn, J. H. (2012). American Society of Clinical Oncology provisional clinical opinion: The integration of palliative care into standard oncology care. *Journal of Clinical Oncology, 30*(8), 880–887. https://doi.org/10.1200/JCO.2011.38.5161.

Soto, G. J., Martin, G. S., & Gong, M. N. (2013). Healthcare disparities in critical illness. *Critical Care Medicine, 41*(12). https://doi.org/10.1097/CCM.0b013e3182a84a43.

Steinhauser, K. E., Clipp, E. C., McNeilly, M., Christakis, N. A., McIntyre, L. M., & Tulsky, J. A. (2000). In search of a good death: Observations of patients, families, and providers. *Annals of Internal Medicine, 132*(10), 825. https://doi.org/10.7326/0003-4819-132-10-200005160-00011.

Teno, J. M., Freedman, V. A., Kasper, J. D., Gozalo, P., & Mor, V. (2015). Is care for the dying improving in the United States? *Journal of Palliative Medicine, 18*(8), 662–666. https://doi.org/10.1089/jpm.2015.0039.

Teno, J. M., Gozalo, P. L., Bynum, J. P. W., Leland, N. E., Miller, S. C., Morden, N. E., Scupp, T., Goodman, D. C., & Mor, V. (2013). Change in end-of-life care for Medicare beneficiaries: Site of death, place of care, and health care transitions in 2000, 2005, and 2009. *Journal of the American Medical Association, 309*(5), 470. https://doi.org/10.1001/jama.2012.207624.

Teno, J. M., Gozalo, P. L., Lee, I. C., Kuo, S., Spence, C., Connor, S. R., & Casarett, D. J. (2011). Does hospice improve quality of care for persons dying from dementia? *Journal of the American Geriatrics Society, 59*(8), 1531–1536. https://doi.org/10.1111/j.1532-5415.2011.03505.x.

Teno, J. M., Mitchell, S. L., Kuo, S. K., Gozalo, P. L., Rhodes, R. L., Lima, J. C., & Mor, V. (2011). Decision-making and outcomes of feeding tube insertion: A five-state study. *Journal of the American Geriatrics Society, 59*(5), 881–886. https://doi.org/10.1111/j.1532-5415.2011.03385.x.

Tieu, L., Schillinger, D., Sarkar, U., Hoskote, M., Hahn, K. J., Ratanawongsa, N., Ralston, J. D., & Lyles, C. R. (2017). Online patient websites for electronic health record access among vulnerable populations: Portals to nowhere? *Journal of the American Medical Informatics Association, 24*(e1), e47–e54. https://doi.org/10.1093/jamia/ocw098.

Timmermans, S. (2005). Death brokering: Constructing culturally appropriate deaths. *Sociology of Health & Illness, 27*(7), 993–1013. https://doi.org/10.1111/j.1467-9566.2005.00467.x.

Tschirhart, E. C., Du, Q., & Kelley, A. S. (2014). Factors influencing the use of intensive procedures at the end of life. *Journal of the American Geriatrics Society, 62*(11), 2088–2094. https://doi.org/10.1111/jgs.13104.

Wachterman, M. W., Pilver, C., Smith, D., Ersek, M., Lipsitz, S. R., & Keating, N. L. (2016). Quality of end-of-life care provided to patients with different serious illnesses. *Journal of the American Medical Association Internal Medicine, 176*(8), 1095–1102. https://doi.org/10.1001/jamainternmed.2016.1200.

Weissman, J. S., Cooper, Z., Hyder, J. A., Lipsitz, S., Jiang, W., Zinner, M. J., & Prigerson, H. G. (2016). End-of-life care intensity for physicians, lawyers, and the general population. *Journal of the American Medical Association, 315*(3), 303–305. https://doi.org/10.1001/jama.2015.17408.

Wohleber, A. M., McKitrick, D. S., & Davis, S. E. (2012). Designing research with hospice and palliative care populations. *American Journal of Hospice and Palliative Medicine, 29*(5), 335–345. https://doi.org/10.1177/1049909111427139.

Wong, S. P. Y., Kreuter, W., & O'Hare, A. M. (2012). Treatment intensity at the end of life in older adults receiving long-term dialysis. *Archives of Internal Medicine, 172*(8), 661–663. https://doi.org/10.1001/archinternmed.2012.268.

Yennurajalingam, S., Noguera, A., Parsons, H. A., Torres-Vigil, I., Duarte, E. R., Palma, A., Bunge, S., Palmer, J. L., Delgado-Guay, M. O., & Bruera, E. (2013). Family caregiver preferences for patient decisional control among Hispanics in the United States and Latin America. *Palliative Medicine, 27*(7), 692–698. https://doi.org/10.1177/0269216313486953.

Yun, Y. H., Kwon, Y. C., Lee, M. K., Lee, W. J., Jung, K. H., Do, Y. R., Kim, S., Heo, D. S., Choi, J. S., & Park, S. Y. (2010). Experiences and attitudes of patients with terminal cancer and their family caregivers toward the disclosure of terminal illness. *Journal of Clinical Oncology, 28*(11), 1950–1957. https://doi.org/10.1200/JCO.2009.22.9658.

4

CARE FOR THE DYING

A key aspect of the predictable death is that patients experience a lengthy period of illness and disability before they die, and so providing and receiving care comprises a significant part of the life course. The average 65-year-old man can expect a year and a half of life with severe disability in his future; the average 65-year-old woman, three years (Freedman et al., 2016). An average young adult may expect to provide unpaid elder care for five years; for some young adults, unpaid care will become their principal occupation for much of the life course (Carmichael & Ercolani, 2016; National Academies of Sciences, Engineering, and Medicine et al., 2016).

Thus, in this chapter, I focus on the people who deliver daily care to dying persons. Some are paid care workers, such as the certified nurse's aides who work in nursing homes. Others are unpaid care workers, such as friends and family. The health care system could not operate without either of these types of workers, and I address both groups here. I explain who comprises both groups, the nature of their working conditions, and the problems and rewards they encounter in caring for dying persons. For paid care workers, I describe the social disparities that immigrants to the U.S. experience, and for unpaid care workers, I describe social disparities by gender.

Care Work

Providing care is part of being a responsible and loving family member in almost all cultures (Piercy, 1998). Adult children feel and express an obligation to care for their parents (Stein et al., 1998), and married people perceive providing care to be an inherent aspect of one's marital relationship (Feeney & Hohaus, 2001). Further, caring can be an intrinsically rewarding experience, with care workers reporting closer relationships, the feeling of doing meaningful work, an increased sense of self-efficacy, and other benefits (Kramer, 1997). Family members of dying persons are especially likely to feel that their care work is meaningful (Waldrop et al., 2005). Therefore, the pervasiveness of low-paying and unpaid long-term care in the U.S. may seem natural and appropriate: The common term *caregiving* itself implies that care is something a person gives freely, donates, or volunteers without expectation of extrinsic reward.

Emphasizing care as an act of love or a good deed can have the effect of de-emphasizing the ways in which care is difficult and valuable work. Care work and other jobs in which people perform work for their family members, or while acting "like family," are often treated as distinct from the capitalist market (Dodson & Zincavage, 2007). Nevertheless, U.S. families live their lives in a capitalist market, and that market does not reward time spent providing care. Such emphasis keeps pay low and job conditions poor in all of the care professions, including long-term care for older and dying persons, child care work, teaching, and nursing (Zelizer, 2005). Such emphasis prevents the labor of stay-at-home parents and eldercare providers from counting as work in the formal economy, for example, towards one's work history in Social Security (Herd, 2006).

Indeed, a distinction between family care and labor market work plays a major role in sustaining the long-term care system that oversees predictable deaths in the U.S., preventing it from having to address questions of just labor practices and the feminization of poverty (Folbre, 2002; Harrington Meyer & Herd, 2007). As Evelyn Nakano Glenn (2012) argues in her book *Forced to care*:

> [T]he social organization of care has been rooted in diverse forms of coercion that have induced women to assume responsibility for caring for family members and that have tracked poor, racial minority, and immigrant women into positions entailing caring for others. The forms of coercion have varied in degree, directness, and explicitness but nonetheless have served to constrain and direct women's choices; the net consequence of restricted choice has been to keep caring labor "cheap," that is, free (in the case of family care labor) or low waged (in the case of paid care labor).
>
> *(p. 5)*

Glenn goes on to identify coercion in gender and familial obligations and in the service labor force, whereby people in power, who historically have been White and male, can command the labor of workers, who are often female and persons of color.

Therefore, in this book I use the term *care work* instead of *caregiving* to describe the labor of paid and unpaid carers. This chapter emphasizes cumulative disadvantage among care workers. That is, a person's experiences and circumstances stay with them throughout the life course and have persistent, long-term effects

(DiPrete & Eirich, 2006). For example, delivering unpaid care to parents in midlife raises women's risk of poverty in later life (Wakabayashi & Donato, 2006). Care work is thus one of the life course factors that serves to stratify people by wealth and opportunity, exacerbating inequalities among older adults (Dannefer, 1987; O'Rand, 1996).

Paid Care Work at the End of Life

Paid care workers go by many titles: home health aides, nurses' assistants, personal care attendants, and so on. Collectively, they are known as the direct care workforce, and they comprise 27% of the health care workforce in the United States (Dawson, 2016). By one estimate, they provide 70 to 80% of the care delivered in institutional long-term care settings such as nursing homes (Dawson, 2016; Harmuth & Dyson, 2005). They constitute one of the largest occupational groups in the United States, outnumbering teachers, cashiers, fast food workers, and public safety workers (PHI, 2011).

Almost all – 89% – of paid care workers are women (Institute of Medicine, 2008). Compared to other women in the paid labor force, care workers are disproportionately likely to be Black or Hispanic (vs. White non-Hispanic) or foreign born (Smith & Baughman, 2007). Over half – 55% – have a high-school education or less (PHI, 2011). Paid care workers are disproportionately likely to be single mothers, which is significant because 44% of married women obtain their health insurance through being their husband's dependent, and single women lack this access (Sohn, 2015). Therefore, approximately one in five paid care workers has no health insurance, and another one in five receives Medicaid (Campbell, 2017). The Affordable Care Act reduced the number of uninsured paid care workers from 28% in 2009, mostly through extension of Medicaid benefits, but lack of insurance is still significantly more common among care workers than among workers in other sectors. Approximately half of paid care workers live below 200% of the poverty line, making them eligible in most states for public assistance in affording food, housing, energy, and child care (PHI, 2013).

Paid care workers are in high demand. As the Baby Boomers age, care work is one of the fastest growing occupations in the United States (PHI, 2013). The insufficient number of care workers is already affecting the quality of care that older persons receive. Nursing homes must turn away prospective patients, and home care recipients experience high levels of unmet need, because there are not enough workers to deliver their care (Graham, 2017). Moreover, there will be an acute shortage of young and midlife women to take new jobs in care. By one estimate, there will be 1.3 million new care jobs by 2022, yet only 227,000 women aged 25 to 54 will have entered the labor force – and many of those women will take other jobs (Dawson, 2016). To fill the positions, the profession will need to attract workers in addition to poor single women of color.

Further, the profession will need to retain current care workers. Turnover is surprisingly difficult to measure (Barry et al., 2008), but sources agree that most care workers stay in their job only for a period of months (Institute of Medicine, 2008). Turnover produces inconsistencies in care, and adversely affects its quality (Castle & Engberg, 2007).

The major cause of shortage of workers and turnover in the workforce is that workload is high, while pay and training are very low in these jobs (Stone & Harahan, 2010). First, care workers have more work than they can do, insufficient assistance with tasks that require multiple workers, and responsibility for large amounts of regulatory paperwork (Cherry et al., 2007). Much of the work is physically demanding, involving lifting and moving patients and assisting them with bathing and toileting. In 2006, there were 526 serious work-related injuries per 10,000 care workers, making it one of the occupations with the highest rates of injury (Bureau of Labor Statistics, 2007). The Bureau of Labor Statistics figure is likely an underestimate, given that there is no way of recording injuries to the approximately 800,000 care workers who work directly for an individual client, rather than an agency or institution (Institute of Medicine, 2008).

Second, compensation is low in care work. Paradoxically, as the demand for care workers has risen, the pay has actually decreased (Dawson, 2016). In 2014, the average hourly wage was $10.85 per hour, down from $11.82 in 2004. Home health service jobs in the Southeastern U.S. pay the worst, often below $9 per hour (United States Government Accountability Office, 2016). To compound this problem, many care jobs are part-time, and they do not come with health insurance, retirement accounts, or other benefits such as paid sick leave or paid vacation. Despite low pay, care workers see their work as a vocation and they develop personal relationships with care recipients (Mittal et al., 2009). Care work is intrinsically rewarding and meaningful, but it is the lack of extrinsic reward that drives women to quit: These are simply not jobs that workers can afford to keep (J. C. Morgan et al., 2013).

Third, most care workers receive little training before they begin the job. Certainly, little is required: At the federal level, some job categories such as nurse's aide require 75 hours of training, while others, such as home health aide, require none at all (Institute of Medicine, 2008). These standards have not changed for 20 years (PHI, 2018). The federal standards for training in dog grooming are higher (Institute of Medicine, 2008). States vary in their own requirements, with 17 requiring more hours than the federal minimum, but only six require the 120 hours that experts suggest (PHI, 2018). Perhaps accordingly, workers report that their employers do not trust them, do not offer them discretion in or autonomy over their work, and do not allow them to contribute their expertise towards patients' care plans (Bowers et al., 2003; Mittal et al., 2009).

Training is particularly sparse with regard to delivering care to dying people (Bamonti et al., 2019; Ewen et al., 2016). Approximately 70% of care workers feel unprepared to care for dying persons (Mohlman et al., 2018). Nevertheless, care workers are often the first people to recognize that patients are close to death, and they grieve when their patients die (Black & Rubinstein, 2005; Boerner et al., 2015). Their grief often goes unrecognized both by employers and by patients' families. Sometimes care workers only learn that a patient has died when they are directed to take the body to the morgue, or when they enter a room to find an empty bed or even a new patient in the bed (Barooah et al., 2015). Some employers have explicit policy that prevents care workers from having any communication with the patient's family after the death (Boerner et al., 2016). Subsequently, care workers are at risk of experiencing burnout, including physical and emotional exhaustion and feelings of depersonalization (Bamonti et al., 2019; Boerner et al., 2017).

Some employers have begun to respond to care workers' need for training and support in caring for dying patients. Some employers provide education in hospice and palliative care (Head et al., 2013; Kelly et al., 2008). Many nursing homes are beginning to recognize that care workers benefit from grief and bereavement support as well as practical skill-building (Chahal et al., 2015). Some interventions provide peer-to-peer support (Vis et al., 2016), some provide spiritual support (Holland & Neimeyer, 2005), and others follow the hospice model by treating care workers as among the people surrounding the patient who require their own care and support (Riesenbeck et al., 2015).

Disparities in Paid Care Work by Nativity

Immigrant women are particularly likely to be paid care workers. In 2014, approximately a quarter of U.S. care workers were foreign born (United States Government Accountability Office, 2016). Comparatively, only 17% of members of the overall labor force were foreign born (Bureau of Labor Statistics, 2019). In some states, such as New York and California, immigrants comprise more than 40% of paid care workers, and in some metropolitan areas, such as New York City and Miami, they comprise more than 70% of such workers (Espinoza, 2018; Hess & Henrici, 2013). Care jobs are easy for migrant women to obtain because of the demand for workers, because the work does not require extensive training, and – for those who are undocumented – because work arrangements are often informal.

The problems that affect all paid care workers are magnified for migrant workers, and they face a unique set of problems as well. First, although pay and benefits are poor for all care workers, nationwide, pay is lowest among care workers who are not citizens (Hartmann & Hayes, 2017). Immigrant care workers work more hours for less money than do native born care workers, and they experience more job strain (Hurtado et al., 2012). Pay and benefits are especially important to non-citizens and to newly naturalized citizens, because they are ineligible for forms of public assistance such as Medicaid.

Language is a second barrier for a large number of migrant care workers. Although about 20% speak only English, another 25% speak English poorly or not at all (Espinoza, 2018). Lack of English fluency can pose problems in communicating with patients and with employers, in obtaining jobs with better working conditions and pay, and so on. The federal government, through the Workforce Innovation and Opportunity Act, provides states with grants to make English language and literacy courses available to citizens and non-citizens who have visas to work in the U.S., provided that they have lived in the U.S. continuously for at least five years. Often based in city or community colleges, these programs combine career training and job placement services with English language training (Henrici, 2013). The most successful programs assist students with tuition, child care, and transportation as well. However, the five-year residency requirement sharply limits the number of immigrants who have access to these programs. Moreover, new public charge rules permit the government to deny citizenship to applicants whose records suggest that they may become future users of public assistance programs (U.S. Citizenship and Immigration Services, 2020).

A third problem facing immigrant care workers concerns legal status. About half of foreign-born care workers have become naturalized U.S. citizens, and half are not citizens (Hartmann & Hayes, 2017). Temporary visas cover agricultural and seasonal workers, highly trained workers with specialized skills, and students and other visitors, but none of these categories apply to care work. Further, temporary work visas are generally tied to a specific position, and losing or changing jobs means losing, or at least having to change, one's visa. Permanent work visas for people without higher education are limited in number annually, and further, quotas apply to sending countries. A woman from Mexico or the Philippines may wait eight years to get one (Hess & Henrici, 2013). For these reasons, most immigrant care workers who are not citizens are in the U.S. on a family-sponsored visa unrelated to work, or they are undocumented. Perhaps 20% of immigrant care workers are undocumented (P. G. Chen et al., 2013; Hess & Henrici, 2013).

Lack of English language knowledge and legal status put immigrant care workers at great risk (Hall & Greenman, 2015). Employers, especially of care workers who work in private homes, can easily abuse and exploit migrant workers, and it is very difficult for the workers to escape these situations (Hondagneu-Sotelo, 2007). For example, a report on care workers at the U.S.–Mexico border told the story of Claudia, a migrant woman who cared for an older woman with advanced dementia (Burnham et al., 2018). The older woman's children irregularly paid Claudia her wage of $200 per week, and Claudia was forced to use her wage to purchase her client's food and medications. Migrant workers have few legal protections, and little means of discovering what legal protections do exist. Further, they have few resources or alternatives (Meghani, 2015). Therefore, if told to or asked to do extra unpaid work, workers will usually do the work rather than risk job loss or even deportation (Stacey, 2005).

Unpaid Care Work at the End of Life

Each year, upwards of 40 million unpaid workers, mostly family members, deliver 37 billion hours of care to older adults, and that this care has a market value of 470 billion dollars (Reinhard et al., 2015). Clearly, the effort necessary to replace these carers with a system of paid workers would be gargantuan. The U.S. government has historically preferred to offer support, instead of pay, to care workers, through provisions in Medicare and Medicaid law, unpaid family and medical leave from employment, and tax credits (Bunis, 2019; Commission on Long-Term Care, 2013). These supports are rather minimal: For example, the Family and Medical Leave Act is written such that at least a quarter of unpaid care workers cannot take advantage of it, either because their employer is not bound by the law or because the care worker is supporting someone – such as an in-law – who does not render an employee eligible for leave (Mayer, 2013).

As with paid care workers, most unpaid care workers are women.[1] Only one-third of unpaid care workers are men, and the modal care worker is the daughter, daughter-in-law, or stepdaughter of the care recipient (National Academies of Sciences, Engineering, and Medicine et al., 2016). Being a care worker alters one's life course trajectories of marriage, childbearing, residence, and employment, as one juggles competing priorities (Barnett, 2013). For example, three-quarters of unpaid care workers live with the care recipient, making care an inescapable full-time job (Wolff et al., 2018).

Unpaid care workers do the same work that paid care workers do; however, they face that work from a unique set of circumstances. First, most have even less medical training than paid care workers have. This situation may be acceptable for carers who help with household chores and with activities of daily living such as bathing and dressing, but these are hardly the only things that care workers do. Modern medicine enables patients who would once have died not only to remain alive, but also to live at home, even if they have intensive care needs. Patients live at home, in non-sterile environments, with open wounds and pressure sores, IV lines, catheters, ventilators, feeding tubes, and dialysis machinery (Moorman & Macdonald, 2013). A quarter of care workers help care recipients manage five or more medications (Donelan et al., 2002). Even teenagers are unpaid care workers who help the older adults in their households to manage complex medication regimens (Nickels et al., 2018). Often, unpaid care workers essentially replace skilled medical professionals (Guberman et al., 2005). Unpaid care workers sometimes have the assistance of paid care workers, but most unpaid care workers do not use the formal support services that are available (Wolff et al., 2007, 2018).

Hospitals take advantage of home medical technologies to offload care and return patients to their homes (Arras & Dubler, 1994; Donelan et al., 2002; Guberman et al., 2005). There are no clear clinical standards for which patients should be in the hospital and which can be safely sent home, nor for how to prepare patients and unpaid care workers to be at home (Lewarski & Gay, 2007;

Sunwoo et al., 2014). Significant minorities of unpaid care workers report receiving no instructions, and those who do receive instruction often receive nothing more than a demonstration at the hospital or a single home visit from a nurse (Donelan et al., 2002).

Health care professionals recognize that care workers need more training to deliver complex care at home, because the treatments are not simple to administer (Lehoux, 2004), and because things go wrong (Bee et al., 2009; Hitchings et al., 2010). Forty percent of home ventilator failures are mechanical problems that have nothing to do with human error (King, 2012). Accidents such as falls and infections happen as well (Masotti et al., 2010). Further, unpaid care workers do make errors: For example, 12% report being aware that they made a mistake in administering medications in the past year (Donelan et al., 2002). These problems are more common in home settings than they are in traditional medical settings (Meyer-Massetti et al., 2018).

A second unique circumstance for unpaid care workers is that they are related to, or very emotionally close to, their care recipients. In comparison, physicians and other medical professionals are strongly discouraged from caring for family members, because the relationship may cloud their judgment (F. M. Chen et al., 2001). Indeed, there is a great deal of literature on stress and strain among unpaid care workers, much of it stemming from the close, personal relationships between care provider and care recipient. Spouses report especially high levels of distress and burden in caring for one another (Pinquart & Sörensen, 2011). Illness and disability alter long marital patterns of interdependency and support, and can entail considerable socioemotional and interpersonal losses for both partners, especially when the ill partner has a degenerative condition such as dementia (Quinn et al., 2009). Additionally, illness and disability can represent new elements in the old dynamics of a marriage: Spousal care workers who had low marital quality before they began to care are often the care workers who suffer the most burden and distress (Steadman et al., 2007). Some researchers suggest that marital therapy can be an effective intervention for distressed spousal care workers (Tough et al., 2017).

Prior relationship quality affects care workers' functioning when the care worker is an adult child, as well (Fauth et al., 2012). The parent–adult child relationship also changes when care becomes necessary, with parents and children negotiating roles that are reversed to some degree (Bastawrous et al., 2014). Further, caring for a parent can place strain on the care worker's other important relationships, such as marriage (Kang & Marks, 2016), with potentially different consequences for husbands and wives (Polenick et al., 2017). Sets of siblings also may have conflicts over the degree to which care work for parents is equally or equitably shared, and this tension is often related to the ways in which family relationships functioned before the parent's need for care (Ingersoll-Dayton et al., 2003; Suitor et al., 2014).

Death and dying put strains on caring relationships that are somewhat distinct from the strains of caring for someone who is not dying. Approximately three-quarters of people who die having at least one unpaid care worker at the time of death, and unpaid care work can become more intensive, with the average decedent receiving 66 hours of unpaid care per week in the last year of life (Ornstein et al., 2017; Rhee et al., 2009; Wolff et al., 2007). Death usually ends a long term of caring for someone who has become increasingly sick and disabled over a period of years, yet perhaps up to a quarter of unpaid care workers say they were not prepared for the person's death (Hebert et al., 2006).

Others experience anticipatory grief before the death that may make the job of care provision even more difficult (Holley & Mast, 2009). The distress of anticipatory grief can impair care workers' decision-making and problem solving (Fowler et al., 2013). Further, high levels of anticipatory grief among care workers can make adjustment after the loss more difficult as well (Burton et al., 2006; Nielsen et al., 2016). Care workers experience some practical relief after the patient dies and the demands of care work cease, but anticipatory grieving does not prevent or lessen grief following the death (Bond et al., 2003; Keene & Prokos, 2008).

Disparities in Unpaid Care Work by Gender

In situations in which there are multiple people who could potentially provide unpaid care to an older person, it is usually a woman who assumes the responsibility (Grigoryeva, 2017). Even though recent cohorts of women have stronger attachments to the paid labor force than did older women, there have been no corresponding declines in a woman's likelihood of providing intense care (i.e., 9 or more hours per week) (Pavalko & Wolfe, 2016). When men do serve as unpaid care workers, their experience is not the same as women's. Men who are care workers provide care for fewer hours than women do, especially in the years before retirement (Glauber, 2017; Henz, 2010). As that finding implies, women disproportionately provide more intense care, such as care for the dying (T. Morgan et al., 2016). Moreover, women have more negative experiences in care work, and thus experience more distress and poorer physical health, than do men in care work (Lin et al., 2012; Swinkels et al., 2019).

The disproportionate experience of unpaid care work has a range of effects on women's lives, but here I focus on how it affects women's finances. Unpaid care work reduces lifetime earnings disproportionately for women. Employed women earn, on average, less than their male counterparts in the same jobs (Institute for Women's Policy Research, 2019). Partly, this gap is because women incur a wage penalty for providing unpaid care that has remained stable across cohorts, while men incur no such penalty (Glauber, 2019). Although such conduct is illegal, many employers discriminate against care workers (Williams et al., 2012). Explicit workplace policies that are friendly to care workers do help women stay in the workforce, but the average employed woman care worker has a job with less access to supervisor support, paid leave, and flexible scheduling than the average employed man care worker (Lahaie et al., 2013; Pavalko & Henderson, 2006).

Sixty percent of employed unpaid care workers report that they need to come in late or leave early, take a leave of absence, or reduce hours at their paid job in order to fulfill their care responsibilities (National Academies of Sciences, Engineering, and Medicine et al., 2016). Care workers often must pass up promotions or other opportunities to advance, such as further education, that those who are not providing care can take (Lilly et al., 2007).

Many care workers need to stop paid employment entirely, because their workplace is not flexible, or because their working income is insufficient to purchase care to replace their own. Thus, among women, care workers are significantly less likely to work for pay than women who do not provide care, although there is no such association for men (Lee & Tang, 2015). Approximately one in five retirees say that they retired in order to provide unpaid care (Helman et al., 2015).

Making a return to the paid labor force after having provided unpaid care can be a challenge, such that the end of a care work role does not predict increasing one's hours in or returning to the paid labor force (Austen & Ong, 2010; Gonzales et al., 2017). Employers do not recognize years spent providing unpaid care as productive time, but rather as a gap in one's resume. Further, care work exacts a toll on physical health, and poor health reduces the likelihood of working for pay (Carson, 2018). One estimate is that a woman aged 62 or older who has been providing care full-time has only a 1–2% chance of receiving a full-time job offer in the next year (Skira, 2015).

Reduced lifetime earnings translate into reduced private pension, savings, and Social Security benefits in retirement. Social Security benefits are based on a person's most lucrative 20 years of paid work, and currently, Social Security does not count unpaid care as work. Social Security is intended to supplement retirees' personal savings and employer pensions, yet over half of single older women earn 90% or more of their income from Social Security (Hartmann et al., 2011). Current Social Security policy assumes married, heterosexual, male-breadwinner families, where the wife's benefit derives from her husband's work history (Harrington Meyer & Herd, 2007). With increasing rates of non-marriage and divorce, fewer women today, especially Black women, can rely on this equation (Harrington Meyer et al., 2005).

Thus, one estimate is that women who are unpaid care workers forgo $324,044 in lost wages and retirement benefits, while men forgo $283,716 (Metropolitan Life Insurance Company, 2011). Losses are especially high for women whose educational attainment and skills are low, a fact that exacerbates the effects of a trend whereby lower-income women are more likely than higher-income women to assume an unpaid care work role (Lee et al., 2015; Wakabayashi & Donato, 2005). Even, further compounding the problem, 30% of unpaid care workers spend money from their personal savings, and 16% spend money that they intended for their own retirement (Rainville et al., 2016). Women in poverty in later life are twice as likely to have provided care to their parents compared to older women who have incomes above the poverty line (Wakabayashi & Donato, 2006).

Summary

A consequence of the predictable death from non-communicable, chronic illnesses is that people require long-term care, sometimes for decades, before they die. U.S. policy lags behind the changes of epidemiological transition, and thus there are not integrated systems to provide long-term care. Future demographic changes – including the aging of the Baby Boomers, lower fertility rates, and increasing proportions of women obtaining higher education and entering the paid labor force – make it unlikely that the supply of care workers will be sufficient to meet the demand for care. The status quo is unsustainable and requires reforms urgently.

The sector of the paid labor force that provides long-term care is called direct care work. Paid care workers are in high demand, yet wages have been declining and even full-time jobs rarely include benefits. The jobs require little educational attainment, and federal requirements mandate 75 hours – or less, for some positions – of job training. Thus, the workers in these jobs are disproportionately poor women of color, often immigrants to the United States. On top of the other problems in the industry, migrant workers face problems with low English language literacy and with their legal status. A particular challenge in care work for dying patients is that there is little emotional support for grieving workers, who may develop close relationships with patients before they die.

Family members and friends also deliver unpaid care that has approximately 500 billion dollars of market worth annually. The federal and state governments do not compensate this work in terms of taxes, Social Security, and paid leave, however. Consequently, providing unpaid care has substantial economic consequences for carers, especially women, in their own later lives.

Note

1. In fact, many paid care workers do double duty, also caring for their own family members each day outside of their paid shift.

References

Arras, J. D., & Dubler, N. N. (1994). Bringing the hospital home: Ethical and social implications of high-tech home care. *The Hastings Center Report*, *24*(5), S19–S28. https://doi.org/10.2307/3563510.

Austen, S., & Ong, R. (2010). The employment transitions of mid-life women: Health and care effects. *Ageing & Society*, *30*(2), 207–227. https://doi.org/10.1017/S0144686X09990511.

Bamonti, P., Conti, E., Cavanagh, C., Gerolimatos, L., Gregg, J., Goulet, C., Pifer, M., & Edelstein, B. (2019). Coping, cognitive emotion regulation, and burnout in long-term care nursing staff: A preliminary study. *Journal of Applied Gerontology*, *38*(1), 92–111. https://doi.org/10.1177/0733464817716970.

Barnett, A. E. (2013). Pathways of adult children providing care to older parents. *Journal of Marriage and Family*, *75*(1), 178–190. https://doi.org/10.1111/j.1741-3737.2012.01022.x.

Barooah, A., Boerner, K., van Riesenbeck, I., & Burack, O. R. (2015). Nursing home practices following resident death: The experience of certified nursing assistants. *Geriatric Nursing, 36*(2), 120–125. https://doi.org/10.1016/j.gerinurse.2014.11.005.

Barry, T., Kemper, P., & Brannon, S. D. (2008). Measuring worker turnover in long-term care: Lessons from the better jobs better care demonstration. *The Gerontologist, 48*(3), 394–400. https://doi.org/10.1093/geront/48.3.394.

Bastawrous, M., Gignac, M. A., Kapral, M. K., & Cameron, J. I. (2014). Daughters providing poststroke care: Perspectives on the parent–child relationship and well-being. *Qualitative Health Research, 24*(11), 1527–1539. https://doi.org/10.1177/1049732314548689.

Bee, P. E., Barnes, P., & Luker, K. A. (2009). A systematic review of informal caregivers' needs in providing home-based end-of-life care to people with cancer. *Journal of Clinical Nursing, 18*(10), 1379–1393. https://doi.org/10.1111/j.1365-2702.2008.02405.x.

Black, H. K., & Rubinstein, R. L. (2005). Direct care workers' response to dying and death in the nursing home: A case study. *The Journals of Gerontology: Series B, 60*(1), S3–S10. https://doi.org/10.1093/geronb/60.1.S3.

Boerner, K., Burack, O. R., Jopp, D. S., & Mock, S. E. (2015). Grief after patient death: Direct care staff in nursing homes and homecare. *Journal of Pain and Symptom Management, 49*(2), 214–222. https://doi.org/10.1016/j.jpainsymman.2014.05.023.

Boerner, K., Gleason, H., & Barooah, A. (2016). Home health aides' experience with client death: The role of employer policy. *Home Healthcare Now, 34*(4), 189–195. https://doi.org/10.1097/NHH.0000000000000360.

Boerner, K., Gleason, H., & Jopp, D. (2017). Burnout after patient death: Challenges for direct care workers. *Journal of Pain and Symptom Management, 54*(3), 317–325. https://doi.org/10.1016/j.jpainsymman.2017.06.006.

Bond, M. J., Clark, M. S., & Davies, S. (2003). The quality of life of spouse dementia caregivers: Changes associated with yielding to formal care and widowhood. *Social Science & Medicine, 57*(12), 2385–2395. https://doi.org/10.1016/S0277-9536(03)00133-3.

Bowers, B. J., Esmond, S., & Jacobson, N. (2003). Turnover reinterpreted: CNAs talk about why they leave. *Journal of Gerontological Nursing, 29*(3), 36–43. https://doi.org/10.3928/0098-9134-20030301-09.

Bunis, D. (2019). *Caregiving tax credit proposal for working families*. AARP. www.aarp.org/caregiving/financial-legal/info-2017/credit-for-caring-act.html.

Bureau of Labor Statistics. (2007). *Nonfatal occupational injuries and illnesses requiring days away from work, 2006* (No. 07–1741).

Bureau of Labor Statistics. (2019). *Foreign-born workers: Labor force characteristics 2018*. www.bls.gov/news.release/forbrn.nr0.htm/Labor-Force-Characteristics-of-Foreign-Born-Workers-Summary.

Burnham, L., Moore, L., & Ohia, E. (2018). *Living in the shadows: Latina domestic workers in the Texas–Mexico border region*. National Domestic Workers Alliance. https://actionnetwork.org/user_files/user_files/000/024/054/original/Living_in_the_Shadows_rpt_Eng_final_screen_(1)_(1).pdf.

Burton, A. M., Haley, W. E., & Small, B. J. (2006). Bereavement after caregiving or unexpected death: Effects on elderly spouses. *Aging & Mental Health, 10*(3), 319–326. https://doi.org/10.1080/13607860500410045.

Campbell, S. (2017). *The impact of the ACA on health coverage for direct care workers*. PHI. https://phinational.org/resource/the-impact-of-the-affordable-care-act-on-health-coverage-for-direct-care-workers/.

Carmichael, F., & Ercolani, M. G. (2016). Unpaid caregiving and paid work over life-courses: Different pathways, diverging outcomes. *Social Science & Medicine, 156*, 1–11. https://doi.org/10.1016/j.socscimed.2016.03.020.

Carson, J. A. (2018). The complexities of family health: Predicting women's employment. *Journal of Family Issues, 39*(5), 1326–1347. https://doi.org/10.1177/0192513X17710281.

Castle, N. G., & Engberg, J. (2007). The influence of staffing characteristics on quality of care in nursing homes. *Health Services Research, 42*(5), 1822–1847. https://doi.org/10.1111/j.1475-6773.2007.00704.x.

Chahal, J. K., Ewen, H. H., Anderson, K., & Miles, T. P. (2015). Institutional bereavement care for fictive kin: Staff grief in CCRCs. *Journal of the American Medical Directors Association, 16*(10), 892–895. https://doi.org/10.1016/j.jamda.2015.06.013.

Chen, F. M., Feudtner, C., Rhodes, L. A., & Green, L. A. (2001). Role conflicts of physicians and their family members: Rules but no rulebook. *Western Journal of Medicine, 175*(4), 236–239.

Chen, P. G., Auerbach, D. I., Muench, U., Curry, L. A., & Bradley, E. H. (2013). Policy solutions to address the foreign-educated and foreign-born health care workforce in the United States. *Health Affairs, 32*(11), 1906–1913. https://doi.org/10.1377/hlthaff.2013.0576.

Cherry, B., Ashcraft, A., & Owen, D. (2007). Perceptions of job satisfaction and the regulatory environment among nurse aides and charge nurses in long-term care. *Geriatric Nursing, 28*(3), 183–192. https://doi.org/10.1016/j.gerinurse.2007.01.015.

Commission on Long-Term Care. (2013). *Report to the Congress*. www.govinfo.gov/content/pkg/GPO-LTCCOMMISSION/pdf/GPO-LTCCOMMISSION.pdf.

Dannefer, D. (1987). Aging as intracohort differentiation: Accentuation, the Matthew effect, and the life course. *Sociological Forum, 2*(2), 211–236. https://doi.org/10.1007/BF01124164.

Dawson, S. L. (2016). The direct care workforce – Raising the floor of job quality. *Generations, 40*(1), 38–46.

DiPrete, T. A., & Eirich, G. M. (2006). Cumulative advantage as a mechanism for inequality: A review of theoretical and empirical developments. *Annual Review of Sociology, 32*(1), 271–297. https://doi.org/10.1146/annurev.soc.32.061604.123127.

Dodson, L., & Zincavage, R. M. (2007). "It's like a family:" Caring labor, exploitation, and race in nursing homes. *Gender & Society, 21*(6), 905–928. https://doi.org/10.1177/0891243207309899.

Donelan, K., Hill, C. A., Hoffman, C., Scoles, K., Feldman, P. H., Levine, C., & Gould, D. (2002). Challenged to care: Informal caregivers in a changing health system. *Health Affairs, 21*(4), 222–231. https://doi.org/10.1377/hlthaff.21.4.222.

Espinoza, R. (2018). *Immigrants and the direct care workforce*. PHI. https://phinational.org/resource/immigrants-and-the-direct-care-workforce-2018/.

Ewen, H. H., Nikzad-Terhune, K., & Chahal, J. K. (2016). The rote administrative approach to death in senior housing: Using the other door. *Geriatric Nursing, 37*(5), 360–364. https://doi.org/10.1016/j.gerinurse.2016.05.003.

Fauth, E., Hess, K., Piercy, K., Norton, M., Corcoran, C., Rabins, P., Lyketsos, C., & Tschanz, J. (2012). Caregivers' relationship closeness with the person with dementia predicts both positive and negative outcomes for caregivers' physical health and psychological well-being. *Aging & Mental Health, 16*(6), 699–711. https://doi.org/10.1080/13607863.2012.678482.

Feeney, J. A., & Hohaus, L. (2001). Attachment and spousal caregiving. *Personal Relationships, 8*(1), 21–39. https://doi.org/10.1111/j.1475-6811.2001.tb00026.x.

Folbre, N. (2002). *The invisible heart: Economics and family values.* The New Press.
Fowler, N. R., Hansen, A. S., Barnato, A. E., & Garand, L. (2013). Association between anticipatory grief and problem solving among family caregivers of persons with cognitive impairment. *Journal of Aging and Health, 25*(3), 493–509. https://doi.org/10.1177/0898264313477133.
Freedman, V. A., Wolf, D. A., & Spillman, B. C. (2016). Disability-free life expectancy over 30 years: A growing female disadvantage in the U.S. population. *American Journal of Public Health, 106*(6), 1079–1085. https://doi.org/10.2105/AJPH.2016.303089.
Glauber, R. (2017). Gender differences in spousal care across the later life course. *Research on Aging, 39*(8), 934–959. https://doi.org/10.1177/0164027516644503.
Glauber, R. (2019). The wage penalty for parental caregiving: Has it declined over time? *Journal of Marriage and Family, 81*(2), 415–433. https://doi.org/10.1111/jomf.12555.
Glenn, E. N. (2012). *Forced to care: Coercion and caregiving in America.* Harvard University Press.
Gonzales, E., Lee, Y., & Brown, C. (2017). Back to work? Not everyone. Examining the longitudinal relationships between informal caregiving and paid work after formal retirement. *The Journals of Gerontology: Series B, 72*(3), 532–539. https://doi.org/10.1093/geronb/gbv095.
Graham, J. (2017). Severe shortage of home health workers robs thousands of proper care. *Kaiser Health News.* https://khn.org/news/severe-shortage-of-home-health-workers-robs-thousands-of-proper-care/.
Grigoryeva, A. (2017). Own gender, sibling's gender, parent's gender: The division of elderly parent care among adult children. *American Sociological Review, 82*(1), 116–146. https://doi.org/10.1177/0003122416686521.
Guberman, N., Gagnon, É., Côté, D., Gilbert, C., Thivièrge, N., & Tremblay, M. (2005). How the trivialization of the demands of high-tech care in the home is turning family members into para-medical personnel. *Journal of Family Issues, 26*(2), 247–272. https://doi.org/10.1177/0192513X04270208.
Hall, M., & Greenman, E. (2015). The occupational cost of being illegal in the United States: Legal status, job hazards, and compensating differentials. *Social Forces, 49*(2), 406–442. https://doi.org/10.1111/imre.12090.
Harmuth, S., & Dyson, S. (2005). *Results of the 2005 national survey of state initiatives on the long-term care direct-care workforce.* National Clearinghouse on the Direct Care Workforce. https://phinational.org/wp-content/uploads/legacy/clearinghouse/RESULTS%20OF%20THE%202005%20NATIONAL%20SURVEY%20FINAL%2092205.pdf.
Harrington Meyer, M., & Herd, P. (2007). *Market friendly or family friendly? The state and gender inequality in old age.* Russell Sage Foundation.
Harrington Meyer, M., Wolf, D. A., & Himes, C. L. (2005). Linking benefits to marital status: Race and Social Security in the U.S. *Feminist Economics, 11*(2), 145–162. https://doi.org/10.1080/13545700500115977.
Hartmann, H., & Hayes, J. (2017). The growing need for home care workers: Improving a low-paid, female-dominated occupation and the conditions of its immigrant workers. *Public Policy & Aging Report, 27*(3), 88–95. https://doi.org/10.1093/ppar/prx017.
Hartmann, H., Hayes, J., & Drago, R. (2011). *Social Security: Especially vital to women and people of color, men increasingly reliant.* Institute for Women's Policy Research. https://iwpr.org/publications/social-security-especially-vital-to-women-and-people-of-color-men-increasingly-reliant/.

Head, B. A., Washington, K. T., & Myers, J. (2013). Job satisfaction, intent to stay, and recommended job improvements: The palliative nursing assistant speaks. *Journal of Palliative Medicine, 16*(11), 1356–1361. https://doi.org/10.1089/jpm.2013.0160.

Hebert, R. S., Dang, Q., & Schulz, R. (2006). Preparedness for the death of a loved one and mental health in bereaved caregivers of patients with dementia: Findings from the REACH study. *Journal of Palliative Medicine, 9*(3), 683–693. https://doi.org/10.1089/jpm.2006.9.683.

Helman, R., Copeland, C., & VanDerhei, J. (2015). *The 2015 retirement confidence survey: Having a retirement savings plan a key factor in Americans' retirement confidence.* Employee Benefit Research Institute. www.ebri.org/content/the-2015-retirement-confidence-survey-having-a-retirement-savings-plan-a-key-factor-in-americans-retirement-confidence-5513.

Henrici, J. (2013). *Improving career opportunities for immigrant women in-home care workers.* Institute for Women's Policy Research. https://iwpr.org/publications/improving-career-opportunities-for-immigrant-women-in-home-care-workers/.

Henz, U. (2010). Parent care as unpaid family labor: How do spouses share? *Journal of Marriage and Family, 72*(1), 148–164. https://doi.org/10.1111/j.1741-3737.2009.00689.x.

Herd, P. (2006). Crediting care or marriage? Reforming Social Security family benefits. *The Journals of Gerontology: Series B, 61*(1), S24–S34. https://doi.org/10.1093/geronb/61.1.S24.

Hess, C., & Henrici, J. M. (2013). *Increasing pathways to legal status for immigrant in-home care workers.* Institute for Women's Policy Research. https://iwpr.org/publications/increasing-pathways-to-legal-status-for-immigrant-in-home-care-workers/.

Hitchings, H., Best, C., & Steed, I. (2010). Home enteral tube feeding in older people: Consideration of the issues. *British Journal of Nursing, 19*(18), 1150–1154. https://doi.org/10.12968/bjon.2010.19.18.79046.

Holland, J. M., & Neimeyer, R. A. (2005). Reducing the risk of burnout in end-of-life care settings: The role of daily spiritual experiences and training. *Palliative & Supportive Care, 3*(3), 173–181. https://doi.org/10.1017/S1478951505050297.

Holley, C. K., & Mast, B. T. (2009). The impact of anticipatory grief on caregiver burden in dementia caregivers. *The Gerontologist, 49*(3), 388–396. https://doi.org/10.1093/geront/gnp061.

Hondagneu-Sotelo, P. (2007). *Domestica: Immigrant workers cleaning and caring in the shadows of affluence.* University of California Press.

Hurtado, D. A., Sabbath, E. L., Ertel, K. A., Buxton, O. M., & Berkman, L. F. (2012). Racial disparities in job strain among American and immigrant long-term care workers. *International Nursing Review, 59*(2), 237–244. https://doi.org/10.1111/j.1466-7657.2011.00948.x.

Ingersoll-Dayton, B., Neal, M. B., Ha, J., & Hammer, L. B. (2003). Redressing inequity in parent care among siblings. *Journal of Marriage and Family, 65*(1), 201–212. https://doi.org/10.1111/j.1741-3737.2003.00201.x.

Institute for Women's Policy Research. (2019). *Pay equity & discrimination.* https://iwpr.org/issue/employment-education-economic-change/pay-equity-discrimination/.

Institute of Medicine. (2008). The direct-care workforce. In *Retooling for an aging America: Building the health care workforce.* National Academies Press. www.ncbi.nlm.nih.gov/books/NBK215393/.

Kang, S., & Marks, N. F. (2016). Marital strain exacerbates health risks of filial caregiving: Evidence from the 2005 National Survey of Midlife in the United States. *Journal of Family Issues, 37*(8), 1123–1150. https://doi.org/10.1177/0192513X14526392.

Keene, J. R., & Prokos, A. H. (2008). Widowhood and the end of spousal care-giving: Relief or wear and tear? *Ageing & Society*, *28*(4), 551–570. https://doi.org/10.1017/S0144686X07006654.

Kelly, K., Ersek, M., Virani, R., Malloy, P., & Ferrell, B. (2008). End-of-life nursing education consortium geriatric training program: Improving palliative care in community geriatric care settings. *Journal of Gerontological Nursing*, *34*(5), 28–35. https://doi.org/10.3928/00989134-20080501-06.

King, A. C. (2012). Long-term home mechanical ventilation in the United States. *Respiratory Care*, *57*(6), 921–932. https://doi.org/10.4187/respcare.01741.

Kramer, B. J. (1997). Gain in the caregiving experience: Where are we? What next? *The Gerontologist*, *37*(2), 218–232. https://doi.org/10.1093/geront/37.2.218.

Lahaie, C., Earle, A., & Heymann, J. (2013). An uneven burden: Social disparities in adult caregiving responsibilities, working conditions, and caregiver outcomes. *Research on Aging*, *35*(3), 243–274. https://doi.org/10.1177/0164027512446028.

Lee, Y., & Tang, F. (2015). More caregiving, less working: Caregiving roles and gender difference. *Journal of Applied Gerontology*, *34*(4), 465–483. https://doi.org/10.1177/0733464813508649.

Lee, Y., Tang, F., Kim, K. H., & Albert, S. M. (2015). The vicious cycle of parental caregiving and financial well-being: A longitudinal study of women. *The Journals of Gerontology: Series B*, *70*(3), 425–431. https://doi.org/10.1093/geronb/gbu001.

Lehoux, P. (2004). Patients' perspectives on high-tech home care: A qualitative inquiry into the user-friendliness of four technologies. *BMC Health Services Research*, *4*(1), 28. https://doi.org/10.1186/1472-6963-4-28.

Lewarski, J. S., & Gay, P. C. (2007). Current issues in home mechanical ventilation. *Chest*, *132*(2), 671–676. https://doi.org/10.1378/chest.07-0558.

Lilly, M. B., Laporte, A., & Coyte, P. C. (2007). Labor market work and home care's unpaid caregivers: A systematic review of labor force participation rates, predictors of labor market withdrawal, and hours of work. *The Milbank Quarterly*, *85*(4), 641–690. https://doi.org/10.1111/j.1468-0009.2007.00504.x.

Lin, I.-F., Fee, H. R., & Wu, H.-S. (2012). Negative and positive caregiving experiences: A closer look at the intersection of gender and relationship. *Family Relations*, *61*(2), 343–358. https://doi.org/10.1111/j.1741-3729.2011.00692.x.

Masotti, P., McColl, M. A., & Green, M. (2010). Adverse events experienced by homecare patients: A scoping review of the literature. *International Journal for Quality in Health Care*, *22*(2), 115–125. https://doi.org/10.1093/intqhc/mzq003.

Mayer, G. (2013). *The family and medical leave act (FMLA): Policy issues* (CRS-R43214). Congressional Research Service. www.dtic.mil/docs/citations/ADA590349.

Meghani, Z. (2015). Trapped in a web of immigration and employment laws: Female undocumented home health workers in the U.S. In *Women migrant workers: Ethical, political and legal problems*. Taylor & Francis. https://doi.org/10.4324/9781315677262-3.

Metropolitan Life Insurance Company. (2011). *MetLife study of caregiving costs to working caregivers*. www.aarp.org/livable-communities/learn/health-wellness/info-12-2012/metlife-study-caregiving-costs-working.html.

Meyer-Massetti, C., Meier, C. R., & Guglielmo, B. J. (2018). The scope of drug-related problems in the home care setting. *International Journal of Clinical Pharmacy*, *40*(2), 325–334. https://doi.org/10.1007/s11096-017-0581-9.

Mittal, V., Rosen, J., & Leana, C. (2009). A dual-driver model of retention and turnover in the direct care workforce. *The Gerontologist*, *49*(5), 623–634. https://doi.org/10.1093/geront/gnp054.

Mohlman, W. L., Dassel, K., Supiano, K. P., & Caserta, M. (2018). End-of-life education and discussions with assisted living certified nursing assistants. *Journal of Gerontological Nursing, 44*(6), 41–48. https://doi.org/10.3928/00989134-20180327-01.

Moorman, S. M., & Macdonald, C. (2013). Medically complex home care and caregiver strain. *The Gerontologist, 53*(3), 407–417. https://doi.org/10.1093/geront/gns067.

Morgan, J. C., Dill, J., & Kalleberg, A. L. (2013). The quality of healthcare jobs: Can intrinsic rewards compensate for low extrinsic rewards? *Work, Employment and Society, 27*(5), 802–822. https://doi.org/10.1177/0950017012474707.

Morgan, T., Williams, L. A., Trussardi, G., & Gott, M. (2016). Gender and family caregiving at the end-of-life in the context of old age: A systematic review. *Palliative Medicine, 30*(7), 616–624. https://doi.org/10.1177/0269216315625857.

National Academies of Sciences, Engineering, and Medicine, Eden, J., Adults, C. on F. C. for O., Services, B. on H. C., Division, H. and M., & National Academies of Sciences, E. (2016). *Families caring for an aging America*. National Academies Press. www.ncbi.nlm.nih.gov/books/NBK396409/.

Nickels, M., Siskowski, C., Lebron, C. N., & Belkowitz, J. (2018). Medication administration by caregiving youth: An inside look at how adolescents manage medications for family members. *Journal of Adolescence, 69*, 33–43. https://doi.org/10.1016/j.adolescence.2018.09.001.

Nielsen, M. K., Neergaard, M. A., Jensen, A. B., Bro, F., & Guldin, M.-B. (2016). Do we need to change our understanding of anticipatory grief in caregivers? A systematic review of caregiver studies during end-of-life caregiving and bereavement. *Clinical Psychology Review, 44*, 75–93. https://doi.org/10.1016/j.cpr.2016.01.002.

O'Rand, A. M. (1996). The precious and the precocious: Understanding cumulative disadvantage and cumulative advantage over the life course. *The Gerontologist, 36*(2), 230–238. https://doi.org/10.1093/geront/36.2.230

Ornstein, K. A., Kelley, A. S., Bollens-Lund, E., & Wolff, J. L. (2017). A national profile of end-of-life caregiving in the United States. *Health Affairs, 36*(7), 1184–1192. https://doi.org/10.1377/hlthaff.2017.0134.

Pavalko, E. K., & Henderson, K. A. (2006). Combining care work and paid work: Do workplace policies make a difference? *Research on Aging, 28*(3), 359–374. https://doi.org/10.1177/0164027505285848.

Pavalko, E. K., & Wolfe, J. D. (2016). Do women still care? Cohort changes in U.S. women's care for the ill or disabled. *Social Forces, 94*(3), 1359–1384. https://doi.org/10.1093/sf/sov101.

PHI. (2011). *Who are direct-care workers?* https://phinational.org/wp-content/uploads/legacy/clearinghouse/PHI%20Facts%203.pdf.

PHI. (2013). *America's direct care workforce*. https://phinational.org/wp-content/uploads/legacy/phi-facts-3.pdf.

PHI. (2018). *Home health aide training requirements by state*. https://phinational.org/advocacy/home-health-aide-training-requirements-state-2016/.

Piercy, K. W. (1998). Theorizing about family caregiving: The role of responsibility. *Journal of Marriage and Family, 60*(1), 109–118. https://doi.org/10.2307/353445.

Pinquart, M., & Sörensen, S. (2011). Spouses, adult children, and children-in-law as caregivers of older adults: A meta-analytic comparison. *Psychology and Aging, 26*(1), 1–14. https://doi.org/10.1037/a0021863.

Polenick, C. A., Seidel, A. J., Birditt, K. S., Zarit, S. H., & Fingerman, K. L. (2017). Filial obligation and marital satisfaction in middle-aged couples. *The Gerontologist, 57*(3), 417–428. https://doi.org/10.1093/geront/gnv138.

Quinn, C., Clare, L., & Woods, B. (2009). The impact of the quality of relationship on the experiences and wellbeing of caregivers of people with dementia: A systematic review. *Aging & Mental Health*, *13*(2), 143–154. https://doi.org/10.1080/13607860802459799.

Rainville, C., Skufca, L., & Mehegan, L. (2016). *Family caregivers cost survey: What they spend & what they sacrifice*. AARP. www.aarp.org/research/topics/care/info-2016/family-caregivers-cost-survey.html?CMP=RDRCT-PPI-CAREGIVING-102416.

Reinhard, S., Feinberg, L. F., Choula, R., & Houser, A. (2015). *Valuing the invaluable: 2015 update*. AARP. www.aarp.org/ppi/info-2015/valuing-the-invaluable-2015-update.html.

Rhee, Y., Degenholtz, H. B., Sasso, A. T. L., & Emanuel, L. L. (2009). Estimating the quantity and economic value of family caregiving for community-dwelling older persons in the last year of life. *Journal of the American Geriatrics Society*, *57*(9), 1654–1659. https://doi.org/10.1111/j.1532-5415.2009.02390.x.

Riesenbeck, I. van, Boerner, K., Barooah, A., & Burack, O. R. (2015). Preparedness for resident death in long-term care: The experience of front-line staff. *Journal of Pain and Symptom Management*, *50*(1), 9–16. https://doi.org/10.1016/j.jpainsymman.2015.02.008.

Skira, M. M. (2015). Dynamic wage and employment effects of elder parent care. *International Economic Review*, *56*(1), 63–93. https://doi.org/10.1111/iere.12095.

Smith, K., & Baughman, R. (2007). Caring for America's aging population: A profile of the direct-care workforce. *Monthly Labor Review*, 20–26.

Sohn, H. (2015). Health insurance and risk of divorce: Does having your own insurance matter? *Journal of Marriage and the Family*, 77(4), 982–995. https://doi.org/10.1111/jomf.12195.

Stacey, C. L. (2005). Finding dignity in dirty work: The constraints and rewards of low-wage home care labour. *Sociology of Health & Illness*, *27*(6), 831–854. https://doi.org/10.1111/j.1467-9566.2005.00476.x.

Steadman, P. L., Tremont, G., & Duncan Davis, J. (2007). Premorbid relationship satisfaction and caregiver burden in dementia caregivers. *Journal of Geriatric Psychiatry and Neurology*, *20*(2), 115–119. https://doi.org/10.1177/0891988706298624.

Stein, C. H., Wemmerus, V. A., Ward, M., Gaines, M. E., & Al, E. (1998). "Because they're my parents:" An intergenerational study of felt obligation and parental caregiving. *Journal of Marriage and Family*, *60*(3), 611. https://doi.org/10.2307/353532

Stone, R., & Harahan, M. F. (2010). Improving the long-term care workforce serving older adults. *Health Affairs*, *29*(1), 109–115. https://doi.org/10.1377/hlthaff.2009.0554.

Suitor, J. J., Gilligan, M., Johnson, K., & Pillemer, K. (2014). Caregiving, perceptions of maternal favoritism, and tension among siblings. *The Gerontologist*, *54*(4), 580–588. https://doi.org/10.1093/geront/gnt065.

Sunwoo, B.Y., Mulholland, M., Rosen, I. M., & Wolfe, L. F. (2014). The changing landscape of adult home noninvasive ventilation technology, use, and reimbursement in the United States. *Chest*, *145*(5), 1134–1140. https://doi.org/10.1378/chest.13-0802.

Swinkels, J., Tilburg, T. van, Verbakel, E., & Broese van Groenou, M. (2019). Explaining the gender gap in the caregiving burden of partner caregivers. *The Journals of Gerontology: Series B*, 74(2), 309–317. https://doi.org/10.1093/geronb/gbx036.

Tough, H., Brinkhof, M. W., Siegrist, J., & Fekete, C. (2017). Subjective caregiver burden and caregiver satisfaction: The role of partner relationship quality and reciprocity. *Archives of Physical Medicine and Rehabilitation*, *98*(10), 2042–2051. https://doi.org/10.1016/j.apmr.2017.02.009.

United States Government Accountability Office. (2016). *Long-term care workforce: Better information needed on nursing assistants, home health aides, and other direct care workers*. www.gao.gov/products/GAO-16-718.

U.S. Citizenship and Immigration Services. (2020, January 30). *USCIS announces public charge rule implementation following Supreme Court stay of nationwide injunctions*. www.uscis.gov/news/news-releases/uscis-announces-public-charge-rule-implementation-following-supreme-court-stay-nationwide-injunctions.

Vis, J.-A., Ramsbottom, K., Marcella, J., McAnulty, J., Kelley, M. L., Kortes-Miller, K., & Jones-Bonofiglio, K. (2016). Developing and implementing peer-led intervention to support staff in long-term care homes manage grief. *SAGE Open*, *6*(3), 2158244016665888. https://doi.org/10.1177/2158244016665888.

Wakabayashi, C., & Donato, K. M. (2005). The consequences of caregiving: Effects on women's employment and earnings. *Population Research and Policy Review*, *24*(5), 467–488. https://doi.org/10.1007/s11113-005-3805-y.

Wakabayashi, C., & Donato, K. M. (2006). Does caregiving increase poverty among women in later life? Evidence from the Health and Retirement survey. *Journal of Health and Social Behavior*, *47*(3), 258–274. https://doi.org/10.1177/002214650604700305.

Waldrop, D. P., Kramer, B. J., Skretny, J. A., Milch, R. A., & Finn, W. (2005). Final transitions: Family caregiving at the end of life. *Journal of Palliative Medicine*, *8*(3), 623–638. https://doi.org/10.1089/jpm.2005.8.623.

Williams, J. C., Devaux, R., Petrac, P., & Feinberg, L. (2012). *Protecting family caregivers from employment discrimination*. AARP. www.aarp.org/content/dam/aarp/research/public_policy_institute/health/protecting-caregivers-employment-discrimination-insight-AARP-ppi-ltc.pdf.

Wolff, J. L., Dy, S. M., Frick, K. D., & Kasper, J. D. (2007). End-of-life care: Findings from a national survey of informal caregivers. *Archives of Internal Medicine*, *167*(1), 40–46. https://doi.org/10.1001/archinte.167.1.40.

Wolff, J. L., Mulcahy, J., Huang, J., Roth, D. L., Covinsky, K., & Kasper, J. D. (2018). Family caregivers of older adults, 1999–2015: Trends in characteristics, circumstances, and role-related appraisal. *The Gerontologist*, *58*(6), 1021–1032. https://doi.org/10.1093/geront/gnx093.

Zelizer, V. (2005). *The purchase of intimacy*. Princeton University Press.

5
SOCIAL ISOLATION

Because long-term, progressive chronic illnesses are the causes of predictable deaths, older people often experience years of moderate to severe disability before death (Freedman et al., 2016). A person diagnosed with Alzheimer's disease, for example, may live with it for up to 20 years (Alzheimer's Association, 2020). Disability often limits individuals' opportunities for social engagement, leaving them socially isolated (Rosso et al., 2013). Technological advances in communication and transportation have created more opportunity for interpersonal connection than ever before, yet one view is that these aspects of modernity actually serve to isolate people by making family and community more voluntary and less accessible (Parigi & Henson, 2014). For example, today's adults aged 18–24 spend more time at home than older groups of adults do, perhaps because they are digital natives who do many daily tasks, even shopping for groceries, online (Todd, 2019).

This chapter will address specifically how isolation is itself a risk factor for early mortality, and why older, less healthy people are particularly at risk of isolation at the end of life (Cornwell & Waite, 2009; Holt-Lunstad, 2018). In the second part of the chapter, I use data from the National Health and Aging Trends Study (NHATS) to describe several different measures of social isolation and then test whether they are associated with the probability of mortality and the quality of death. These results reveal new information about social isolation broadly as a fundamental cause of health outcomes, as well as new information about the extent to which individuals can use their social resources to improve their own death quality.

Social Isolation at the End of Life

Social connection has all four of the essential features necessary to be called a fundamental cause of health inequality: It is a flexible resource that can be used to affect multiple risk factors for multiple causes of death enduringly over historical time (Phelan et al., 2010).[1] Like other fundamental causes, social engagement is a resource people can use to maintain good health, while social isolation is a risk factor for early mortality, with causes ranging from suicide to heart disease and stroke (Chu et al., 2017; Valtorta et al., 2016). In fact, social isolation is a stronger predictor of mortality than better-known factors such as obesity (Holt-Lunstad et al., 2015). The reasons why are numerous and complex: Engagement with others supplies physical exercise, social support, a sense of purpose, encouragement to engage in healthy behaviors, assistance in visiting the doctor and following his or her prescribed course of treatment, and numerous other health benefits (Berkman et al., 2000; Thoits, 2011). I will not attempt to exhaustively review the mechanisms here. In keeping with my emphasis on social disparities, I will simply note the dynamic interplay between social isolation and health status, where people in poor health are disproportionately likely to be socially isolated, and in turn, social isolation is a cause of physical and cognitive decline (Shankar et al., 2013, 2017).

Social isolation is the objective absence of social ties, while loneliness is the subjective experience of having an insufficient social life (R. S. Weiss, 1973). Often the two co-occur, yet they are distinct phenomena that are independently associated with poor health outcomes (Steptoe et al., 2013). A person may feel lonely despite having social ties, for example if those relationships are negative and a source of strain (Moorman, 2016). At the end of their lives, people are at risk of loneliness even if they are surrounded by others, because the way others treat them changes (Sand & Strang, 2006). Being a dying person is lonely. Spiritual care is important in end of life settings as people cope with the knowledge that their very existence, as we know it, will end (Edwards et al., 2010).

Social Disparities in Social Isolation

Many people think of social engagement as primarily the product of one's own choices. However, social isolation that is systematic and imposed upon people with some level of intentionality is social exclusion or social exclusivity (Agulnik, 2002). In this sense, most people are socially isolated to some degree. For example, most people move through their days within a bubble of people like themselves: Advantaged White people live, work, and do other activities near other advantaged White people, while disadvantaged people of color live, work, and do other activities near other disadvantaged people of color (Krivo et al., 2013). This kind of isolation (or social exclusivity) may be desirable to advantaged White people, who wish to retain their social resources. Yet I argue that social isolation is an inherent problem even here, because it means that advantaged White people lack access to the viewpoints and ideas of people different from themselves, and so do not trust disadvantaged people nor engage in civic groups that would promote social engagement across racial/ethnic and class lines (Kawachi et al., 1997). Further, social isolation intersects with other ways of being marginalized in society such as racism, sexism, or lack of education. Therefore, social disparities in isolation are as important to examine as disparities on the basis of ascribed characteristics like race/ethnicity or gender.

Social isolation is particularly concentrated among people in poor health who have one or more disabilities, for a variety of reasons. One simple reason is that public spaces often lack the physical modifications that can help people navigate safely, such that people who have disabilities may restrict their social participation in order to avoid injury (Denkinger et al., 2015). Other disabilities, such as sensory or cognitive impairments, may pose barriers to communicating with others (Alma et al., 2011; Desrosiers et al., 2009).

Beyond these physical or environmental barriers, disabilities have psychosocial consequences that can result in social isolation. First, depression is a common consequence of developing a disability, and people who are depressed often become socially withdrawn as a symptom of the illness (Yuen et al., 2015). Depression and disability form a vicious cycle, because depression itself is further disabling (Friedrich, 2017). Second, many people with disabilities live in poverty, because disabilities can be costly to treat and can limit participation in the workforce (Drew, 2015). People in poverty are less socially engaged and connected than people with more material resources (Mood & Jonsson, 2016; Samuel et al., 2018; Whittle et al., 2017). Finally, disabilities are stigmatized. Social isolation is perhaps the most prominent consequence of stigma, given that stigma is socially constructed among the person with the stigma, his or her social network members, and complete strangers (Garthwaite, 2015; Livingston & Boyd, 2010; Sherry & Neller, 2016).

Data from the National Health and Aging Trends Study

Next, I conduct an analysis of longitudinal survey data on social engagement among older persons, focusing on the probability of dying. In 2011, Johns Hopkins University, the University of Michigan, and the research corporation Westat began NHATS. They surveyed a random sample of Medicare beneficiaries about their living arrangements and communities, health and mobility, and economic and social well-being. Participants included 7,609 men and women who ranged in age from 65 to over 90 years old. Their sociodemographic characteristics are presented in column two of Table 5.1. Further technical details about the sample and the study design are available in the Data Appendix to this chapter.

NHATS included four different ways to measure levels of social isolation. First, it obtained information on participants' living arrangements, categorizing them as living alone (33%); living with a spouse or partner only (40%); living with a spouse or partner and other persons (9%); and living with other persons only (18%). My interest is in people who live alone versus those who live with any other person. Living alone is a well-established risk factor for mortality in the United States and around the world (Davis et al., 1992; Kandler et al., 2007; Koskinen et al., 2007;

Ng et al., 2015; Pimouguet et al., 2016). Among several different ways in which this type of social isolation can be dangerous is the simple absence of assistance. A fall, a stroke or heart attack, or some otherwise treatable condition may become deadly if a person cannot obtain medical attention promptly (De Luca et al., 2004; Saver et al., 2016). Having another person in the household to call for help is a significant advantage. Additionally, some evidence indicates that older adults who live alone fall more often than older adults who live with others (Elliott et al., 2009). These persons may fall while attempting household tasks, such as climbing ladders, that in other households are done more safely by household members with better balance and visual acuity.

Among NHATS participants, sociodemographic patterns shaped who lived alone or with others, as shown in the right-hand columns of Table 5.1. I examined many of the fundamental causes that I cover in this book: gender, age, educational attainment, race/ethnicity, region of the country, income, and immigrant status. I did not include sexual orientation because NHATS did not ask participants for this information. Nearly three-quarters (73%) of people who lived alone were women, and non-Hispanic White persons were also disproportionately likely to live alone. People who lived alone had much lower average annual incomes than people who lived with others. Factors that protected against living alone included having a four-year college degree or more education, being Hispanic, and being an immigrant to the United States.

Health status is important to measure well when investigating these research questions. That is, if chronic illness or disability is a cause of social isolation, yet the analyses do not account for health, the results may look as though social isolation causes mortality, when in fact poor health alone is the key risk factor. NHATS measured participants' health status very thoroughly, and I include six different measures of health in these analyses. First, participants were asked "Would you say that in general, your health is excellent, very good, good, fair, or poor?" This type of question measures subjective health, which predicts mortality even after accounting for multiple objective measures of health (Idler & Benyamini, 1997). Second, participants were asked if they had had an overnight hospital stay in the past year. Third, participants were asked if they had fallen down in the past year,[2] because falls are associated with increased risk of death and often indicating underlying frailty or osteoporosis (Dunn et al., 1992). Fourth, participants were asked whether a doctor had ever told them that they had a heart attack or myocardial infarction; any heart disease including angina or congestive heart failure; high blood pressure or hypertension; diabetes; lung disease, such as emphysema, asthma, or chronic bronchitis; a stroke; dementia or Alzheimer's Disease; and cancer. I summed these illnesses. Fifth, participants were asked about whether they experienced each of four depressive symptoms not at all, several days in the past month, more than half the days, or nearly every day. These included apathy, hopelessness, anxiousness, and inability to stop worrying. I calculated a mean score for each participant. Finally, participants answered questions about their physical capacity

TABLE 5.1 Characteristics of Participants by Living Arrangements, 2011 National Health and Aging Trends Study, $N=7{,}609$

	Total sample	*Lives with others*	*Lives alone*	*p*
Percent female	58	51	73	***
Age (% per group)				
65–69	19	21	12	***
70–74	21	22	18	***
75–79	20	21	17	***
80–84	20	19	22	**
85–89	13	10	17	***
90+	9	6	14	***
Educational attainment (% per group)				
Less than high school	27	27	27	*ns*
High school graduate	28	27	30	**
Some college	24	24	25	*ns*
BA or more	21	22	17	***
Race/ethnicity (% per group)				
White non-Hispanic	69	68	71	**
Black non-Hispanic	22	21	23	*ns*
Hispanic	6	7	4	***
Other race/ethnicity	3	3	2	**
Region (% per area)				
Northeast	19	18	20	*
Midwest	23	22	26	***
South	39	40	37	*
West	19	20	17	***
Average income ($)	43,366	49,052	31,773	***
Percent foreign-born	11	12	9	***
Self-reported health (1 = excellent; 5 = poor)	2.86 (1.13)	2.84 (1.14)	2.89 (1.10)	*ns*
Hospital stay, past year (%)	23	23	24	*ns*
Fall, past year (%)	23	23	24	*ns*
Number of serious illnesses	1.85 (1.34)	1.86 (1.35)	1.83 (1.31)	*ns*

Notes

ns indicates that the difference between those who live alone and those who live with others is not statistically significant. Asterisks denote statistical significance where $*p<0.05$, $**p<0.01$, $***p<0.001$.

to walk three blocks, climb one flight of stairs, carry a ten pound item, bend over, reach above their heads, and grasp small objects. I summed up the number of motions with which each participant reported problems.

Among NHATS participants, there were relatively few systematic differences in the health of participants who lived alone or with others, as shown in the right-hand columns of Table 5.1. Those who lived alone reported more frequent depressive symptoms and a larger number of physical limitations than people who lived with others. Older adults who lived alone and with others experienced the other health problems at similar rates, perhaps because an exacerbation in a health condition can be a reason why older adults stop living alone (Gaugler et al., 2007). That is, the group of older adults who live alone is a select group of individuals who are healthy enough to manage the tasks of daily life without another person coresident in their home.

The second way to characterize social isolation in the NHATS data is to look at the social network roster, or the set of questions the survey asked about "who you talk to about important things in your life. This may include good or bad things that happen to you, problems you are having, or important concerns you may have." Participants were instructed: "Looking back over the last year, who are the people you talked with most often about important things?" Participants could name up to five confidantes, and they answered questions about each of those persons. The average person named 1.9 confidantes (SD = 1.3).

A small social network is a risk factor for mortality (Becofsky et al., 2015; Shye et al., 1995). A small social network alone, however, does not necessarily indicate social isolation. In the past, gerontologists believed that older adults had little control over the size of their social networks because of the inevitability of losses due to dementia and death. Now, gerontologists have made clear that older adults often choose deliberately to have smaller networks than younger adults (Carstensen et al., 1999). Younger adults have social goals, such as launching a career and building a family, where having lots of social contacts can be beneficial. Older adults tend to have social goals, such as maintaining a positive mood, that are sometimes best served by limiting social contacts to important, meaningful people (Carstensen et al., 2003). Nevertheless, most people do have a network size below which they feel lonely, and a small social network can indicate that a person does not have sufficient social support (McLaughlin et al., 2010).

I focus on the 521 people (7% of the sample) who named no confidante, as compared to participants who named at least one confidante. The sociodemographic and health characteristics of these two groups, as well as the overall sample, are tabulated in Table 5.1B of the Appendix. Most of the sociodemographic characteristics did not distinguish between people who did and did not have confidantes, but there were a few notable differences that marked these socially isolated people as otherwise marginalized. Men comprised 40% of the sample, but 48% of people who named no confidantes. Those with less than a high-school education, Black non-Hispanic participants, and low-income participants were also disproportionately likely to be among those who named no confidantes. In terms of health, people with no network members had poorer self-reports of their health, and a larger number of physical limitations than did people who had at least one confidante.

Family ties are a third way to characterize social isolation in the NHATS. Participants reported whether they had a spouse or non-marital partner and whether they had living children. Nearly half the sample (47%) had both. Another substantial proportion (43%) had no living spouse or partner, but did have adult children. Three percent were married or partnered without children, and 7% had neither partner nor children.

Marriage, in particular, forms a very important buffer against illness and death, especially for men (Rogers, 1995). Further, lack of family ties is an important measure of social isolation at the end of life because of the state laws in place to make medical decisions on behalf of dying people who lack decisional capacity. A competent person may appoint almost any adult to make those decisions on his or her behalf, and overwhelmingly a spouse or adult child is the preferred appointee (Carr & Khodyakov, 2007; Moorman & Boerner, 2018). Only about half of participants in NHATS had designated a decision-maker (Harrison et al., 2016). Therefore, many states automatically designate one's next-of-kin, usually a spouse or adult child, to make medical decisions in case of incapacity. This situation leaves older persons without these close family ties at risk of dying after receiving life-prolonging treatment during a long-duration hospital stay (Cohen et al., 2015; B. D. Weiss et al., 2012).

I focus on NHATS participants who do not have a spouse/partner or children, as compared to participants who have at least one immediate family member. The sociodemographic and health characteristics of these two groups, as well as the overall sample, are tabulated in Table 5.1C of the Appendix. Whereas men were disproportionately represented among those without confidantes, women were disproportionately represented among those without immediate kin. Black non-Hispanic persons and those over the age of 90 were also associated with having no immediate family. The average income for people who had no immediate kin was only two-thirds of the average income of those who had a partner or children. These characteristics are consistent with the selective nature of getting, and staying, married: Wealthy White people are more likely to marry than are poorer people of color, while female gender and older age are associated with becoming widowed (Horn et al., 2013; Sasson & Umberson, 2014). Older adults residing in the Northeastern U.S. were least likely to report having immediate family. People without immediate family had *fewer* serious diagnoses, but also more physical limitations, than people who had a partner and/or children.

The fourth and final way to measure social isolation in this study is through reports of social participation. Participants were asked whether in the last month they had: (a) visited in person with friends or family not living with you, either at your home or theirs; (b) attended religious services; (c) participated in clubs, classes, or other organized activities besides religious services; and (d) gone out for enjoyment, such as going out to dinner, a movie, to gamble, or to hear music or see a play.

The average person had done 2.3 of those activities (SD=1.3), with 85% having visited family or friends, 58% having attended religious services, 34% having participated in organized activities, and 74% having gone out for enjoyment. However, over 1,000 people (12% of the sample) had done none of these things in the past month.

That social participation protects people against death is now an old finding and one that motivates programming in nursing homes and other long-term care settings (Kiely et al., 2000). Some studies suggest that purposive activities such as education, paid work, or volunteering are most beneficial (Minagawa & Saito, 2015; Okun et al., 2013), while others note the benefits of religious participation (Hummer et al., 1999), and still others show that almost any leisure activity has benefits, with group activities being best (Agahi & Parker, 2008; Fushiki et al., 2012). Scholars are beginning to identify the aspects of activities that matter, such as use of the body and mind, interactions with others, and benefit to others (Chen et al., 2019; Matz-Costa et al., 2016).

I focus on NHATS participants who were socially inactive in the past month, as compared to participants who participated in one or more social activities outside the home. The sociodemographic and health characteristics of these two groups, as well as the overall sample, are tabulated in Table 5.1D of the Appendix. There were strong social gradients between participators and non-participators. The older a person, the less likely he or she was to be socially active. Women were significantly less likely to be active than men were, and the more educational attainment a person had, the more social involvement. For example, 55% of people who were socially inactive had not completed a high-school education. Social inactivity was more common in the Northeastern U.S., less common in the Western U.S., and more common among foreign-born older adults. As with the other types of social isolation, income was significantly lower among socially inactive persons as compared to people who had participated in one or more activities. Further, those who were socially inactive were significantly poorer on every measure of health included in the study. For example, 36% of socially inactive participants had been hospitalized in the past year, compared to only 23% of people who engaged in at least one form of participation. Depressive symptoms and physical limitations were also remarkably high among people who did not participate in any activities.

An interesting question is the extent to which these four forms of social isolation co-occur. This information is shown in Table 5.2. Of the 6,989 people who could be classified on all four measures, 60% were not isolated in any way. Another quarter lived alone, but had confidantes, immediate kin, and social activities. The remaining 15% had a variety of different constellations of isolation and engagement. Only 12 participants were isolated in all four ways, and there were no participants who said that they lived with others but had no confidantes, immediate family, or social activities. This result may indicate the efficacy of group living situations, such as assisted living, at facilitating social activities for interested residents. Living alone and having no spouse or children described 4% of the sample, who may have compensated with confidantes and activities outside the home. Perhaps the 3% of the sample who said that they had others in the household, a spouse and/or children, and activities, but no confidantes, were indicating loneliness. In short, while almost all participants had some type of social involvement, and a majority of participants were not socially isolated in any of the four ways, approximately four in ten participants were isolated in at least one way.

After 2011, NHATS followed up with participants annually, such that by the end of 2017, participants had been interviewed up to seven times. When participants died between interviews, NHATS obtained that information, and where possible, interviewed a proxy respondent who was knowledgeable about the decedent's last month of life. About a quarter of the sample (1,816 people) died by the end of 2017. Thirty-eight percent of the sample remained living and engaged in the study, and another 38% left the study at some point after 2011. (Some participants in this last 38% died and there was no proxy available to complete a last month of life interview, but this situation was rare. At each wave, last month of life interviews were obtained on over 90% of participants who had died in the past year.)

The next step is to estimate whether any of the four forms of social isolation was associated with mortality, net of the sociodemographic composition of the isolated groups and their health status at the beginning of the study. I conducted regression

TABLE 5.2 Co-occurrence of Types of Social Isolation, 2011 National Health and Aging Trends Study, $N = 6{,}989$

Lives alone	*Has no social network members*	*Has no spouse or children*	*No social participation*	*n*	*%*
No	No	No	No	4,172	59.7
Yes	No	No	No	1,760	25.2
Yes	No	Yes	No	250	3.6
No	Yes	No	No	217	3.1
No	No	No	Yes	151	2.2
Yes	Yes	No	No	150	2.2
Yes	No	No	Yes	79	1.1
No	No	Yes	No	73	1.0
Yes	Yes	Yes	No	57	.8
No	Yes	No	Yes	26	.4
Yes	Yes	No	Yes	17	.2
Yes	Yes	Yes	Yes	12	.2
Yes	No	Yes	Yes	11	.2
No	Yes	Yes	No	8	.1
No	No	Yes	Yes	6	.1
No	Yes	Yes	Yes	0	0

analyses. A regression is a type of statistical analysis that allowed me to compare the groups according to their composition on multiple factors simultaneously. Table 5.3 focuses on the differences in social isolation between people who died and people who remained alive and in the study. Table 5.3A, in the Appendix, shows the complete results of the regression analysis, including differences in sociodemographic characteristics and in health as well as differences in social isolation.

There were two important differences between the social engagement of participants who died and participants who remained in the study, net of other measures of social isolation, participants' sociodemographic characteristics, and health status at the baseline of the study. First, mortality was more likely among unmarried participants, both those who had adult children and those who did not, net of income, race/ethnicity, gender, and age. This result is consistent with a broad literature on the health benefits of marriage and marriage-like relationships, which may persist even after adjusting for the fact that more advantaged, healthier people are the most likely to become and remain married (Rogers, 1995; Sasson & Umberson, 2014). Second, each additional social activity that a participant engaged in in 2011 was associated with 20% lower odds of mortality before the end of 2017. This effect corresponds to a 39% chance of death if one is involved in no activities, compared to a 29% chance if one is involved in four activities.

Finally, I focused on indicators of quality of death among the 1,816 participants who died. I conducted regression analyses for three outcomes, as asked of proxy respondents in the interview about the participant's last month of life. First, interviewees were asked how, overall, they would rate the participant's care in the last month of life. Forty-nine percent rated the care as excellent, 31% rated it as very good, and 20% rated it as good, fair, or poor. Second, proxies reported where the person died. Thirty-five percent died at their own

TABLE 5.3 Abridged Results, Multinomial Logistic Regression, Social Isolation in 2011 as a Predictor of Mortality by 2017, National Health and Aging Trends Study, *N*=7,609

	Odds Ratio (CI)
Lives alone	0.83 (0.69–1.00)
Number of social network members (0–5 persons)	1.00 (0.95–1.06)
Next of kin (reference: married with adult children)	
Married, no children	0.94 (0.60–1.48)
Unmarried, with adult children	1.26* (1.03–1.53)
Unmarried, no children	1.57** (1.15–2.15)
Number of social activities, last month (0–4 activities)	0.80*** (0.75–0.85)

Note
The difference between decedents and survivors is shown. Asterisks denote statistical significance where *$p<0.05$, **$p<0.01$, ***$p<0.001$.

home or the home of a loved one, 32% died in the hospital, and 33% died somewhere else, such as a long-term care or hospice facility. Third, interviewees were asked, "During the last month of the participant's life, was there any decision made about care or treatment that s/he would not have wanted?" Ten percent said that there was a decision that went against the preferences of the dying person.

Table 5.4 shows the social isolation results for three regressions that predicted each of the death quality outcomes. Tables 5.4A through 5.4C in the Appendix show the complete results of the regression analyses for all three outcomes, including social isolation factors, sociodemographic characteristics, and health status. Social isolation had little to do with quality of death among participants who died. The only statistically significant result was that people who lived alone were more likely to die in the hospital than to die at home. Even this result is not necessarily an indicator of a poor quality death: To be able to die at home, patients require strong social support from family and friends (Gomes & Higginson, 2006). Without such support, older adults may find that their needs are better met in a hospital (Pollock, 2015).

These results are broadly consistent with other research that indicates few differences in quality of death experiences by race/ethnicity, gender, and socio-economic status among Medicare beneficiaries in the NHATS study (Luth, 2017) and in studies of other populations (Carr, 2016). These authors suggest that fundamental causes of disparities may have little power to change death quality, because

TABLE 5.4 Abridged Results for Multiple Regressions, Social Isolation in 2011 as a Predictor of Three Indicators of Quality of Death, National Health and Aging Trends Study, *N* = 1,816

	Good/fair/poor care (vs. excellent care)	*Hospital death (vs. home)*	*Any unwanted care (vs. none)*
	Odds Ratio (CI)	*Odds Ratio (CI)*	*Odds Ratio (CI)*
Lives alone	1.21 (0.87–1.68)	1.48* (1.09–2.00)	0.80 (0.52–1.21)
Number of social network members (0–5 persons)	0.97 (0.87–1.09)	1.01 (0.92–1.12)	1.00 (0.87–1.16)
Next of kin (reference: married with adult children)			
Married, no children	1.63 (0.65–4.09)	1.11 (0.49–2.50)	0.75 (0.17–3.28)
Unmarried, with adult children	1.20 (0.83–1.73)	0.92 (0.67–1.28)	1.08 (0.70–1.68)
Unmarried, no children	1.36 (0.77–2.41)	0.96 (0.57–1.61)	0.88 (0.42–1.88)
Number of social activities (0–4 activities)	0.91 (0.80–1.03)	1.07 (0.96–1.19)	0.91 (0.78–1.06)

Note

Each column represents a regression model. Participants died between 2011 and the end of 2017. Asterisks denote statistical significance where $*p < 0.05$

there are not resources one can buy – nor social connections one may make – that will substantially change one's quality of death (Carr, 2016). That is, disparities in a health outcome increase to the extent that the health outcome is under human control, because people who are advantaged in regards to the fundamental causes are able to leverage those advantages for preferable outcomes (Oster, 2018; Phelan & Link, 2005). Issues such as the delivery of unwanted or low-quality care may be so structural and systemic that individual-level resources – such as social engagement – do not help people get better outcomes.

Limitations

There are limitations to the data and analysis that readers should take into account when drawing conclusions. First, although NHATS researchers managed to conduct a last month of life interview for over 90% of decedents, there are some for whom no proxy could be found. These people may have been more socially isolated than decedents who had at least one person who could report confidently on their last month of life. If the most socially isolated people do not appear in the data, the results may be too conservative. Second, while NHATS asked many questions about participants' objective social circumstances, it did not include many questions about how participants felt. There are no questions about loneliness, or quality of relationships, or the sorts of support that people received in their relationships. These subjective elements of people's social relationships may matter for their mortality risk and for their quality of death.

Third, by design, my analyses included baseline measures of both health status and social engagement. These data do not tell us which came first, poor health or social isolation. A more definitively causal design might be to identify healthy but socially isolated participants at baseline and to follow only these individuals across the years. That design would, however, only yield information about healthy but socially isolated people, who might be relatively rare in the general population. All study designs entail strengths and weaknesses.

Future Directions

I conclude with a brief agenda for future research in this area. First, a statistical technique called event history analysis could be employed to test not only whether social isolation increases the probability of mortality, but also whether social isolation shortens the amount of time until one dies. That is, NHATS began in 2011. Some participants had died by 2012, others died each subsequent year, and still others were still alive for the 2017 wave of data collection. Event history analysis maximizes upon that information to identify whether, other things being equal, more socially isolated people died sooner, or perhaps younger, than less socially isolated people.

Second, future studies might examine causes of death, or characteristics of causes of death. This information might account for some of the odder results in this analysis. For example, the more depressive symptoms a person had, the more likely he or she was to die at home, rather than in the hospital. One hypothesis is that dying at home generally happens following a long illness with a predictable course that provides enough time for the patient to become depressed, such as cancer, whereas dying in the hospital may be more likely in the case of an acute health crisis such as a heart attack. Social isolation might contribute to either or both illnesses, but the mechanisms would likely differ.

Third, researchers should further theorize about how to measure social isolation. In this chapter, I focused on types: living alone, lacking immediate family, etc. Perhaps degree may be the more important factor; that is, perhaps I should have summed the number of types of isolation people experienced. Alternately, there may be a threshold or critical value after which adding further social engagement has diminishing returns. For example, if a person is involved in only one activity, adding a second might make a large difference for mortality risk. But if a person is involved in five activities, adding a sixth might have little effect. There may even be an unhealthy degree of social engagement, perhaps for example if one's social ties demand time and energy that a person could be spending on tending his or her health. I have posed this challenge as an issue of measurement in empirical research, but in fact this question is important to public health. If the aim is to reduce mortality through social policies and public organizations that enhance social engagement, then decision-makers need to know what kinds of interventions will be effective and efficient.

Summary

Social isolation – an objective lack of social connections – and loneliness – a subjective desire for more social connection – are associated with morbidity and mortality among older Americans. The order of events is unclear, because sick and disabled people are more likely to become socially isolated than healthy people, but social isolation does hasten death. The National Health and Aging Trends Study measures isolation in terms of living arrangements (i.e., alone vs. with others), number of confidantes, existence of immediate family, and participation in social activities. Included together in a model of mortality, and net of sociodemographic characteristics (e.g., age) and health status, marriage and participation in activities were particularly important protective factors. Among measures of quality of death, however, social isolation was less important. People who lived alone were more likely than others to die in the hospital; otherwise, social isolation was not associated with quality of end-of-life care, the location of death, or whether the decedent received unwanted care.

Data Appendix

NHATS researchers generated a sample from the Medicare enrollment database with the primary aim of studying capacity, the disablement process, and forms of assistance as people age (Freedman, 2009). The enrollment database is an excellent way to sample older Americans, because Medicare is nearly universal: In 2016, 94% of Americans aged 65 and older were enrolled in Medicare (U.S. Census Bureau, 2017). NHATS researchers conducted their sampling in three stages. First, they selected counties in the lower 48 United States, with a selection probability proportionate to the Medicare population size within the county.[3] Second, within sampled counties, NHATS researchers selected zip codes, again with a selection probability proportionate to the Medicare population size within the zip code. Finally, within sampled zip codes, NHATS researchers selected study participants. This time, their random sample was stratified for age group and for race/ethnicity, to ensure that NHATS would have sufficiently large groups of participants in each age group and race/ethnic category for statistical analysis. Results can be rebalanced to look as they would had the study design been a simple random sample; I did not rebalance the results I present here.

Of the beneficiaries invited to participate in the study in 2011, 71% agreed, yielding a sample size of 8,245. The subsample I used for analysis is smaller, at 7,609 participants, because 636 of the participants who lived in residential care settings received a different survey that focused more heavily on the care setting and did not include the questions I analyze here. Once in the study, participants tended to remain. At each wave, over 85% of participants who were still living continued in the study. Response was also very good for the interviews with a proxy respondent following a participant's death: At each wave, last month of life data were collected on over 90% of the participants who had died in the last year.

Notes

1. In the public health literature, scholars use the phrase *social capital* commonly than *social engagement*, but the terms have similar meanings. If ordinarily, *capital* is a financial resource, then *social capital* refers to the ways in which social relationships are resources. The book *Bowling alone: The collapse and revival of American community* (Putnam, 2001) was not the first use of the term *social capital*, but it is probably the work that introduced the idea to most scholars of public health and has most influenced further development of the concept.
2. Falling down was defined as "Any fall, slip, or trip in which you lose your balance and land on the floor or ground or at a lower level."
3. If every county had an equal probability of selection, the sample would be a simple random sample. Accounting for some characteristic, such as population size, and then conducting a random sample is called stratified random sampling. Stratified random sampling preserves the benefits of randomness in the sample while also ensuring that the final sample represents important features of Medicare beneficiaries.

TABLE 5.A1 Characteristics of Participants by Presence of a Social Network, 2011 National Health and Aging Trends Study, $N=7,609$

	Total sample	*At least one social network member*	*No social network members*	*p*
Percent female	58	59	51	***
Age (% per group)				
65–69	19	20	18	*ns*
70–74	21	22	21	*ns*
75–79	20	20	20	*ns*
80–84	20	20	22	*ns*
85–89	13	11	12	*ns*
90+	9	7	7	*ns*
Educational attainment (% per group)				
Less than high school	27	25	32	***
High school graduate	28	28	27	*ns*
Some college	24	25	22	*ns*
BA or more	21	22	19	*ns*
Race/ethnicity (% per group)				
White non-Hispanic	69	71	60	***
Black non-Hispanic	22	21	31	***
Hispanic	6	6	6	*ns*
Other race/ethnicity	3	2	3	*ns*
Region (% per area)				
Northeast	19	19	17	*ns*
Midwest	23	24	24	*ns*
South	39	39	42	*ns*
West	19	19	17	*ns*
Average income ($)	43,366	45,407	34,043	***
Percent foreign-born	11	10	11	*ns*
Self-reported health (1 = excellent; 5 = poor)	2.86 (1.13)	2.80 (1.10)	2.91 (1.17)	*
Hospital stay, past year (%)	23	22	21	*ns*
Fall, past year (%)	23	23	19	*ns*
Number of serious illnesses	1.85 (1.34)	1.79 (1.31)	1.71 (1.35)	*ns*
Depression (1 = none; 4 = most)	1.51 (0.65)	1.47 (0.60)	1.50 (0.68)	*ns*
Number of physical limitations	1.32 (1.85)	1.12 (1.71)	1.33 (1.84)	**

Note

ns indicates that the difference between those who live alone and those who live with others is not statistically significant. Asterisks denote statistical significance where *$p<0.05$, **$p<0.01$, ***$p<0.001$.

TABLE 5.A2 Characteristics of Participants by Presence of Next-of-Kin, 2011 National Health and Aging Trends Study, N=7,609

	Total sample	*Spouse and/or child(ren)*	*No spouse or children*	*p*
Percent female	58	58	67	***
Age (% per group)				
65–69	19	19	16	*ns*
70–74	12	21	18	*ns*
75–79	20	20	14	***
80–84	20	20	23	*ns*
85–89	13	12	15	*ns*
90+	9	8	14	***
Educational attainment (% per group)				
Less than high school	27	27	31	*
High school graduate	28	28	27	*ns*
Some college	24	24	20	**
BA or more	21	21	22	*ns*
Race/ethnicity (% per group)				
White non-Hispanic	69	69	63	**
Black non-Hispanic	22	22	29	***
Hispanic	6	6	4	*ns*
Other race/ethnicity	3	3	3	*ns*
Region (% per area)				
Northeast	19	18	24	***
Midwest	23	23	20	*ns*
South	39	39	40	*ns*
West	19	20	16	*ns*
Average income ($)	43,366	44,444	28,449	***
Percent foreign-born	11	11	9	*ns*
Self-reported health (1=excellent; 5=poor)	2.86 (1.13)	2.86 (1.13)	2.85 (1.08)	*ns*
Hospital stay, past year (%)	23	23	23	*ns*
Fall, past year (%)	23	23	24	*ns*
Number of serious illnesses	1.85 (1.34)	1.87 (1.34)	1.62 (1.23)	***
Depression (1=none; 4=most)	1.51 (0.65)	1.51 (0.65)	1.52 (0.62)	*ns*
Number of physical limitations	1.32 (1.85)	1.29 (1.84)	1.69 (2.02)	***

Note

ns indicates that the difference between those who live alone and those who live with others is not statistically significant. Asterisks denote statistical significance where *$p<0.05$, **$p<0.01$, ***$p<0.001$.

TABLE 5.A3 Characteristics of Participants by Social Participation, 2011 National Health and Aging Trends Study, $N=7,609$

	Total sample	*Any social participation*	*No social participation*	*p*
Percent female	58	58	69	***
Age (% per group)				
65–69	19	19	5	***
70–74	21	21	9	***
75–79	20	20	12	***
80–84	20	20	20	*ns*
85–89	13	12	23	***
90+	9	8	29	***
Educational attainment (% per group)				
Less than high school	27	26	55	***
High school graduate	28	28	21	**
Some college	24	25	15	***
BA or more	21	22	9	***
Race/ethnicity (% per group)				
White non-Hispanic	69	70	66	**
Black non-Hispanic	22	21	26	**
Hispanic	6	6	6	*ns*
Other race/ethnicity	3	3	3	*ns*
Region (% per area)				
Northeast	19	18	24	***
Midwest	23	24	23	*ns*
South	39	39	40	*ns*
West	19	20	13	***
Average income ($)	43,366	44,431	23,279	***
Percent foreign-born	11	11	16	**
Self-reported health (1 = excellent; 5 = poor)	2.86 (1.13)	2.81 (1.11)	3.72 (1.12)	***
Hospital stay, past year (%)	23	23	36	***
Fall, past year (%)	23	23	30	**
Number of serious illnesses	1.85 (1.34)	1.82 (1.32)	2.41 (1.52)	***
Depression (1 = none; 4 = most)	1.51 (0.65)	1.48 (0.62)	2.00 (0.87)	***
Number of physical limitations	1.32 (1.85)	1.21 (1.77)	3.34 (2.17)	***

Note

ns indicates that the difference between those who live alone and those who live with others is not statistically significant. Asterisks denote statistical significance where $*p<0.05$, $**p<0.01$, $***p<0.001$.

TABLE 5.A4 Multinomial Logistic Regression, Social Isolation in 2011 as a Predictor of Mortality by 2017, National Health and Aging Trends Study, N=7,609

	Died, last month of life interview	*Left the study*
	Remained in the study	
	Odds Ratio (CI)	Odds Ratio (CI)
Lives alone	0.83 (0.69–1.00)	0.79** (0.67–0.93)
Number of social network members (0–5 persons)	1.00 (0.95–1.06)	0.95 (0.91–1.00)
Next of kin (reference: married with adult children)		
Married, no children	0.94 (0.60–1.48)	1.05 (0.77–1.42)
Unmarried, with adult children	1.26* (1.03–1.53)	0.99 (0.84–1.17)
Unmarried, no children	1.57** (1.15–2.15)	1.08 (0.83–1.41)
Number of social activities, last month (0–4 activities)	0.80*** (0.75–0.85)	0.89*** (0.84–0.94)
Female	0.60*** (0.51–0.70)	0.88* (0.78–0.99)
Five-year age category (65–69–90+)	1.80*** (1.72–1.90)	1.07** (1.02–1.11)
Educational attainment (reference: high school graduate)		
Less than high school	0.92 (0.77–1.11)	0.85* (0.73–0.99)
Some college	0.96 (0.79–1.16)	0.87 (0.74–1.00)
BA or more	0.75** (0.60–0.92)	0.62*** (0.53–0.73)
Race/ethnicity (reference: White non-Hispanic)		
Black non-Hispanic	0.89 (0.75–1.06)	1.17* (1.02–1.35)
Hispanic	0.65* (0.46–0.93)	1.07 (0.82–1.39)
Other race/ethnicity	0.87 (0.55–1.40)	1.36 (0.97–1.91)
Region (Reference: Northeast)		
Midwest	1.03 (0.84–1.28)	0.64*** (0.54–0.76)
South	0.92 (0.76–1.12)	0.73*** (0.63–0.85)
West	1.31* (1.05–1.63)	0.80** (0.67–0.95)
Average income (natural log)	0.94* (0.88–0.99)	0.94* (0.90–0.99)
Foreign-born	0.80 (0.61–1.05)	1.37** (1.13–1.68)
Self-reported health (1 = excellent; 5 = poor)	1.29*** (1.20–1.39)	1.08* (1.02–1.15)
Hospital stay, past year	1.47*** (1.26–1.72)	0.99 (0.86–1.14)
Fall, past year	1.05 (0.89–1.25)	0.91 (0.79–1.05)
Number of serious illnesses	1.18*** (1.11 1–24)	0.98 (0.94–1.03)
Depression (1 = none; 4 = most; natural log)	1.17 (0.96–1.44)	0.95 (0.80–1.13)
Number of physical limitations (natural log)	1.29** (1.10–1.52)	1.04 (0.91–1.18)

Note
Statistical significance denoted as ***p <0.001; **p <0.01; *p <0.05.

TABLE 5.A5 Multinomial Logistic Regression of Social Isolation in 2011 as a Predictor of Overall End-of-Life Care Quality, National Health and Aging Trends Study, $N=1{,}816$

	Very good care	*Good, fair, or poor care*
	Excellent care	
	Odds Ratio (CI)	*Odds Ratio (CI)*
Lives alone	1.07 (0.81–1.43)	1.21 (0.87–1.68)
Number of social network members (0–5 persons)	0.99 (0.90–1.09)	0.97 (0.87–1.09)
Next of kin (reference: married with adult children)		
Married, no children	1.19 (0.51–2.78)	1.63 (0.65–4.09)
Unmarried, with adult children	1.27 (0.93–1.74)	1.20 (0.83–1.73)
Unmarried, no children	1.46 (0.89–2.39)	1.36 (0.77–2.41)
Number of social activities, last month (0–4 activities)	0.95 (0.86–1.06)	0.91 (0.80–1.03)
Female	1.02 (0.79–1.32)	1.03 (0.78–1.39)
Five-year age category (65–69–90+)	0.95 (0.87–1.03)	0.80** (0.73–0.88)
Educational attainment (reference: high school graduate)		
Less than high school	1.00 (0.75–1.33)	1.01 (0.72–1.43)
Some college	0.90 (0.66–1.23)	1.06 (0.73–1.54)
BA or more	0.62* (0.43–0.90)	0.83 (0.54–1.28)
Race/ethnicity (reference: White non-Hispanic)		
Black non-Hispanic	1.05 (0.77–1.42)	1.50* (1.07–2.11)
Hispanic	1.62 (0.87–3.05)	3.01** (1.55–5.85)
Other race/ethnicity	2.57* (1.21–5.45)	1.14 (0.39–3.38)
Region (Reference: Northeast)		
Midwest	1.43* (1.01–2.04)	1.02 (0.69–1.52)
South	1.50* (1.07–2.10)	0.87 (0.59–1.26)
West	1.45* (1.01–2.10)	1.05 (0.69–1.58)
Average income (natural log)	1.09 (0.99–1.20)	1.02 (0.92–1.14)
Foreign-born	0.78 (0.48–1.25)	0.78 (0.45–1.35)
Self-reported health (1 = excellent; 5 = poor)	0.96 (0.86–1.08)	0.99 (0.86–1.14)
Hospital stay, past year	1.16 (0.91–1.48)	1.13 (0.85–1.49)
Fall, past year	1.02 (0.79–1.32)	1.37 (1.00–1.89)
Number of serious illnesses	0.97 (0.89–1.05)	1.01 (0.92–1.11)
Depression (1 = none; 4 = most; natural log)	1.26 (0.92–1.73)	1.21 (0.84–1.75)
Number of physical limitations (natural log)	0.92 (0.73–1.15)	0.82 (0.63–1.06)

Note
Participants died between 2011 and the end of 2017. Asterisks denote statistical significance where $^{*}p<0.05$, $^{**}p<0.001$.

TABLE 5.A6 Multinomial Logistic Regression of Social Isolation in 2011 as a Predictor of Place of Death, National Health and Aging Trends Study, $N = 1,816$

	Hospital	*Another Place*
	Home	
	Odds Ratio (CI)	*Odds Ratio (CI)*
Lives alone	1.48* (1.09–2.00)	1.54** (1.14–2.07)
Number of social network members (0–5 persons)	1.01 (0.92–1.12)	1.01 (0.90–1.12)
Next of kin (reference: married with adult children)		
Married, no children	1.11 (0.49–2.50)	0.74 (0.30–1.86)
Unmarried, with adult children	0.92 (0.67–1.28)	1.00 (0.72–1.39)
Unmarried, no children	0.96 (0.57–1.61)	1.09 (0.65–1.82)
Number of social activities, last month (0–4 activities)	1.07 (0.96–1.19)	0.96 (0.85–1.07)
Female	0.92 (0.70–1.19)	0.90 (0.69–1.17)
Five-year age category (65–69–90+)	0.93 (0.86–1.01)	1.12** (1.03–1.22)
Educational attainment (reference: high school graduate)		
Less than high school	1.17 (0.86–1.59)	0.92 (0.68–1.25)
Some college	0.95 (0.68–1.32)	0.86 (0.62–1.20)
BA or more	0.85 (0.58–1.25)	0.94 (0.65–1.37)
Race/ethnicity (reference: White non-Hispanic)		
Black non-Hispanic	1.40* (1.02–1.90)	0.92 (0.67–1.27)
Hispanic	1.30 (0.71–2.40)	0.62 (0.31–1.23)
Other race/ethnicity	2.27* (1.01–5.09)	0.88 (0.34–2.33)
Region (Reference: Northeast)		
Midwest	0.84 (0.58–1.22)	0.93 (0.65–1.33)
South	0.89 (0.63–1.26)	0.90 (0.64–1.27)
West	0.75 (0.51–1.08)	0.48*** (0.33–0.70)
Average income (natural log)	1.01 (0.92–1.12)	0.99 (0.89–1.09)
Foreign-born	1.12 (0.67–1.81)	1.16 (0.70–1.91)
Self-reported health (1=excellent; 5=poor)	0.99 (0.88–1.12)	0.89 (0.79–1.01)
Hospital stay, past year	0.84 (0.65 1.09)	0.93 (0.72–1.20)
Fall, past year	1.15 (0.85–1.56)	1.20 (0.92–1.58)
Number of serious illnesses	1.04 (0.95–1.13)	0.98 (0.89–1.07)
Depression (1=none; 4=most; natural log)	0.65** (0.46–0.90)	1.19 (0.86–1.66)
Number of physical limitations (natural log)	0.91 (0.74–1.13)	0.95 (0.76–1.18)

Note
Participants died between 2011 and the end of 2017. Asterisks denote statistical significance where *$p < 0.05$, **$p < 0.01$, ***$p < 0.001$.

TABLE 5.A7 Binary Logistic Regression of Social Isolation in 2011 as a Predictor of Unwanted Care, National Health and Aging Trends Study, $N = 1{,}816$

	Odds Ratio (CI)
Lives alone	0.80 (0.52–1.21)
Number of social network members (0–5 persons)	1.00 (0.87–1.16)
Next of kin (reference: married with adult children)	
Married, no children	0.75 (0.17–3.28)
Unmarried, with adult children	1.08 (0.70–1.68)
Unmarried, no children	0.88 (0.42–1.88)
Number of social activities, last month (0–4 activities)	0.91 (0.78–1.06)
Female	0.79 (0.55–1.15)
Five-year age category (65–69–90+)	0.95 (0.84–1.07)
Educational attainment (reference: high school graduate)	
Less than high school	1.07 (0.70–1.64)
Some college	0.97 (0.60–1.55)
BA or more	1.27 (0.76–2.13)
Race/ethnicity (reference: White non-Hispanic)	
Black non-Hispanic	0.87 (0.56–1.36
Hispanic	1.96 (0.91–4.23)
Other race/ethnicity	0.56 (0.13–2.50)
Region (Reference: Northeast)	
Midwest	0.77 (0.47–1.25)
South	0.71 (0.45–1.12)
West	0.88 (0.53–1.44)
Average income (natural log)	0.96 (0.84–1.10)
Foreign-born	0.84 (0.42–1.68)
Self-reported health (1 = excellent; 5 = poor)	1.05 (0.88–1.24)
Hospital stay, past year	0.66* (0.46–0.94)
Fall, past year	1.48* (1.03–2.12)
Number of serious illnesses	1.23** (1.08–1.37)
Depression (1 = none; 4 = most; natural log)	0.98 (0.62–1.53)
Number of physical limitations (natural log)	0.98 (0.69–1.39)
Hispanic	1.96 (0.91–4.23)
Other race/ethnicity	0.56 (0.13–2.50)
Region (Reference: Northeast)	
Midwest	0.77 (0.47–1.25)
South	0.71 (0.45–1.12)
West	0.88 (0.53–1.44)
Average income (natural log)	0.96 (0.84–1.10)
Foreign-born	0.84 (0.42–1.68)
Self-reported health (1 = excellent; 5 = poor)	1.05 (0.88–1.24)
Hospital stay, past year	0.66* (0.46–0.94)
Fall, past year	1.48* (1.03–2.12)
Number of serious illnesses	1.23** (1.08–1.37)
Depression (1 = none; 4 = most; natural log)	0.98 (0.62–1.53)
Number of physical limitations (natural log)	0.98 (0.69–1.39)

Note
Participants died between 2011 and the end of 2017. Asterisks denote statistical significance where $^{*}p < 0.05$, $^{**}p < 0.001$.

References

Agahi, N., & Parker, M. G. (2008). Leisure activities and mortality: Does gender matter? *Journal of Aging and Health*, *20*(7), 855–871. https://doi.org/10.1177/0898264308324631.

Agulnik, P. (2002). *Understanding social exclusion*. Oxford University Press.

Alma, M. A., Mei, S. F. van der, Melis-Dankers, B. J. M., Tilburg, T. G. van, Groothoff, J. W., & Suurmeijer, T. P. B. M. (2011). Participation of the elderly after vision loss. *Disability and Rehabilitation*, *33*(1), 63–72. https://doi.org/10.3109/09638288.2010.488711.

Alzheimer's Association. (2020). *Stages of Alzheimer's*. https://alz.org/alzheimers-dementia/stages.

Becofsky, K. M., Shook, R. P., Sui, X., Wilcox, S., Lavie, C. J., & Blair, S. N. (2015). Influence of the source of social support and size of social network on all-cause mortality. *Mayo Clinic Proceedings*, *90*(7), 895–902. https://doi.org/10.1016/j.mayocp.2015.04.007.

Berkman, L. F., Glass, T., Brissette, I., & Seeman, T. E. (2000). From social integration to health: Durkheim in the new millennium. *Social Science & Medicine*, *51*(6), 843–857. https://doi.org/10.1016/S0277-9536(00)00065-4.

Carr, D. (2016). Is death "the great equalizer"? The social stratification of death quality in the United States. *The ANNALS of the American Academy of Political and Social Science*, *663*(1), 331–354. https://doi.org/10.1177/0002716215596982.

Carr, D., & Khodyakov, D. (2007). Health care proxies: Whom do young old adults choose and why? *Journal of Health and Social Behavior*, *48*(2), 180–194. https://doi.org/10.1177/002214650704800206.

Carstensen, L. L., Isaacowitz, D. M., & Charles, S. T. (1999). Taking time seriously. A theory of socioemotional selectivity. *The American Psychologist*, *54*(3), 165–181. https://doi.org/10.1037//0003-066x.54.3.165.

Carstensen, L. L., Fung, H. H., & Charles, S. T. (2003). Socioemotional selectivity theory and the regulation of emotion in the second half of life. *Motivation and Emotion*, *27*(2), 103–123. https://doi.org/10.1023/A:1024569803230.

Chen, Y.-C., Putnam, M., Lee, Y. S., & Morrow-Howell, N. (2019). Activity patterns and health outcomes in later life: The role of nature of engagement. *The Gerontologist*, *59*(4), 698–708. https://doi.org/10.1093/geront/gny023.

Chu, C., Buchman-Schmitt, J. M., Stanley, I. H., Hom, M. A., Tucker, R. P., Hagan, C. R., Rogers, M. L., Podlogar, M. C., Chiurliza, B., Ringer-Moberg, F. B., Michaels, M. S., Patros, C., & Joiner, T. E. (2017). The interpersonal theory of suicide: A systematic review and meta-analysis of a decade of cross-national research. *Psychological Bulletin*, *143*(12), 1313–1345. https://doi.org/10.1037/bul0000123.

Cohen, A. B., Wright, M. S., Cooney, L., & Fried, T. (2015). Guardianship and end-of-life decision making. *Journal of the American Medical Association Internal Medicine*, *175*(10), 1687–1691. https://doi.org/10.1001/jamainternmed.2015.3956.

Cornwell, E. Y., & Waite, L. J. (2009). Measuring social isolation among older adults using multiple indicators from the NSHAP study. *The Journals of Gerontology: Series B*, *64B*(suppl_1), i38–i46. https://doi.org/10.1093/geronb/gbp037.

Davis, M. A., Neuhaus, J. M., Moritz, D. J., & Segal, M. R. (1992). Living arrangements and survival among middle-aged and older adults in the NHANES I epidemiologic follow-up study. *American Journal of Public Health*, *82*(3), 401–406. https://doi.org/10.2105/AJPH.82.3.401.

De Luca, G., Suryapranata, H., Ottervanger, J. P., & Antman, E. M. (2004). Time delay to treatment and mortality in primary angioplasty for acute myocardial infarction. *Circulation*, *109*(10), 1223–1225. https://doi.org/10.1161/01.CIR.0000121424.76486.20.

Denkinger, M. D., Lukas, A., Nikolaus, T., & Hauer, K. (2015). Factors associated with fear of falling and associated activity restriction in community-dwelling older adults: A systematic review. *The American Journal of Geriatric Psychiatry*, *23*(1), 72–86. https://doi.org/10.1016/j.jagp.2014.03.002.

Desrosiers, J., Wanet-Defalque, M.-C., Témisjian, K., Gresset, J., Dubois, M.-F., Renaud, J., Vincent, C., Rousseau, J., Carignan, M., & Overbury, O. (2009). Participation in daily activities and social roles of older adults with visual impairment. *Disability and Rehabilitation*, *31*(15), 1227–1234. https://doi.org/10.1080/09638280802532456.

Drew, J. A. R. (2015). Disability, poverty, and material hardship since the passage of the ADA. *Disability Studies Quarterly*, *35*(3). https://doi.org/10.18061/dsq.v35i3.4947.

Dunn, J. E., Rudberg, M. A., Furner, S. E., & Cassel, C. K. (1992). Mortality, disability, and falls in older persons: The role of underlying disease and disability. *American Journal of Public Health*, *82*(3), 395–400. https://doi.org/10.2105/AJPH.82.3.395.

Edwards, A., Pang, N., Shiu, V., & Chan, C. (2010). The understanding of spirituality and the potential role of spiritual care in end-of-life and palliative care: A meta-study of qualitative research. *Palliative Medicine*, *24*(8), 753–770. https://doi.org/10.1177/0269216310375860.

Elliott, S., Painter, J., & Hudson, S. (2009). Living alone and fall risk factors in community-dwelling middle age and older adults. *Journal of Community Health*, *34*(4), 301. https://doi.org/10.1007/s10900-009-9152-x.

Freedman, V. A. (2009). Adopting the ICF language for studying late-life disability: A field of dreams? *The Journals of Gerontology: Series A*, *64A*(11), 1172–1174. https://doi.org/10.1093/gerona/glp095.

Freedman, V. A., Wolf, D. A., & Spillman, B. C. (2016). Disability-free life expectancy over 30 years: A growing female disadvantage in the U.S. population. *American Journal of Public Health*, *106*(6), 1079–1085. https://doi.org/10.2105/AJPH.2016.303089.

Friedrich, M. J. (2017). Depression is the leading cause of disability around the world. *Journal of the American Medical Association*, *317*(15), 1517–1517. https://doi.org/10.1001/jama.2017.3826.

Fushiki, Y., Ohnishi, H., Sakauchi, F., Oura, A., & Mori, M. (2012). Relationship of hobby activities with mortality and frailty among community-dwelling elderly adults: Results of a follow-up study in Japan. *Journal of Epidemiology*, *22*(4), 340–347. https://doi.org/10.2188/jea.JE20110057.

Garthwaite, K. (2015). "Keeping meself to meself" – How social networks can influence narratives of stigma and identity for long-term sickness benefits recipients. *Social Policy & Administration*, *49*(2), 199–212. https://doi.org/10.1111/spol.12119.

Gaugler, J. E., Duval, S., Anderson, K. A., & Kane, R. L. (2007). Predicting nursing home admission in the U.S: A meta-analysis. *BMC Geriatrics*, 7(1), 13. https://doi.org/10.1186/1471-2318-7-13.

Gomes, B., & Higginson, I. J. (2006). Factors influencing death at home in terminally ill patients with cancer: Systematic review. *British Medical Journal*, *332*(7540), 515–521. https://doi.org/10.1136/bmj.38740.614954.55.

Harrison, K. L., Adrion, E. R., Ritchie, C. S., Sudore, R. L., & Smith, A. K. (2016). Low completion and disparities in advance care planning activities among older Medicare beneficiaries. *Journal of the American Medical Association Internal Medicine*, *176*(12), 1872–1875. https://doi.org/10.1001/jamainternmed.2016.6751.

Holt-Lunstad, J. (2018). The potential public health relevance of social isolation and loneliness: Prevalence, epidemiology, and risk factors. *Public Policy & Aging Report*, 27(4), 127–130. https://doi.org/10.1093/ppar/prx030.

Holt-Lunstad, J., Smith, T. B., Baker, M., Harris, T., & Stephenson, D. (2015). Loneliness and social isolation as risk factors for mortality: A meta-analytic review. *Perspectives on Psychological Science, 10*(2), 227–237. https://doi.org/10.1177/1745691614568352.

Horn, E. E., Xu, Y., Beam, C. R., Turkheimer, E., & Emery, R. E. (2013). Accounting for the physical and mental health benefits of entry into marriage: A genetically informed study of selection and causation. *Journal of Family Psychology, 27*(1), 30–41. https://doi.org/10.1037/a0029803.

Hummer, R. A., Rogers, R. G., Nam, C. B., & Ellison, C. G. (1999). Religious involvement and U.S. adult mortality. *Demography, 36*(2), 273–285. https://doi.org/10.2307/2648114.

Idler, E. L., & Benyamini, Y. (1997). Self-rated health and mortality: A review of twenty-seven community studies. *Journal of Health and Social Behavior, 38*(1), 21–37. JSTOR. https://doi.org/10.2307/2955359.

Kandler, U., Meisinger, C., Baumert, J., Löwel, H., & the KORA Study Group. (2007). Living alone is a risk factor for mortality in men but not women from the general population: A prospective cohort study. *BMC Public Health*, 7(1), 335. https://doi.org/10.1186/1471-2458-7-335.

Kawachi, I., Kennedy, B. P., Lochner, K., & Prothrow-Stith, D. (1997). Social capital, income inequality, and mortality. *American Journal of Public Health, 87*(9), 1491–1498. https://doi.org/10.2105/AJPH.87.9.1491.

Kiely, D. K., Simon, S. E., Jones, R. N., & Morris, J. N. (2000). The protective effect of social engagement on mortality in long-term care. *Journal of the American Geriatrics Society, 48*(11), 1367–1372. https://doi.org/10.1111/j.1532-5415.2000.tb02624.x.

Koskinen, S., Joutsenniemi, K., Martelin, T., & Martikainen, P. (2007). Mortality differences according to living arrangements. *International Journal of Epidemiology, 36*(6), 1255–1264. https://doi.org/10.1093/ije/dym212.

Krivo, L. J., Washington, H. M., Peterson, R. D., Browning, C. R., Calder, C. A., & Kwan, M.-P. (2013). Social isolation of disadvantage and advantage: The reproduction of inequality in urban space. *Social Forces, 92*(1), 141–164. https://doi.org/10.1093/sf/sot043.

Livingston, J. D., & Boyd, J. E. (2010). Correlates and consequences of internalized stigma for people living with mental illness: A systematic review and meta-analysis. *Social Science & Medicine, 71*(12), 2150–2161. https://doi.org/10.1016/j.socscimed.2010.09.030.

Luth, E. A. (2017). *Social and health determinants of end-of-life care quality: A multidimensional approach* [Doctoral dissertation]. https://rucore.libraries.rutgers.edu/rutgers-lib/53695/.

Matz-Costa, C., Carr, D. C., McNamara, T. K., & James, J. B. (2016). Physical, cognitive, social, and emotional mediators of activity involvement and health in later life. *Research on Aging, 38*(7), 791–815. https://doi.org/10.1177/0164027515606182.

McLaughlin, D., Vagenas, D., Pachana, N. A., Begum, N., & Dobson, A. (2010). Gender differences in social network size and satisfaction in adults in their 70s. *Journal of Health Psychology, 15*(5), 671–679. https://doi.org/10.1177/1359105310368177.

Minagawa, Y., & Saito, Y. (2015). Active social participation and mortality risk among older people in Japan: Results from a nationally representative sample. *Research on Aging, 37*(5), 481–499. https://doi.org/10.1177/0164027514545238.

Mood, C., & Jonsson, J. O. (2016). The social consequences of poverty: An empirical test on longitudinal data. *Social Indicators Research, 127*(2), 633–652. https://doi.org/10.1007/s11205-015-0983-9.

Moorman, S. M. (2016). Dyadic perspectives on marital quality and loneliness in later life. *Journal of Social and Personal Relationships, 33*(5), 600–618. https://doi.org/10.1177/0265407515584504.

Moorman, S. M., & Boerner, K. (2018). How social network size and quality affect end-of-life surrogate preferences. *The Journals of Gerontology: Series B*. https://doi.org/10.1093/geronb/gbx031.

Ng, T. P., Jin, A., Feng, L., Nyunt, M. S. Z., Chow, K. Y., Feng, L., & Fong, N. P. (2015). Mortality of older persons living alone: Singapore Longitudinal Ageing Studies. *BMC Geriatrics*, *15*(1), 126. https://doi.org/10.1186/s12877-015-0128-7.

Okun, M. A., Yeung, E. W., & Brown, S. (2013). Volunteering by older adults and risk of mortality: A meta-analysis. *Psychology and Aging*, *28*(2), 564–577. https://doi.org/10.1037/a0031519.

Oster, E. (2018). *Behavioral feedback: Do individual choices influence scientific results?* [National Bureau of Economic Research Working Paper]. National Bureau of Economic Research. https://doi.org/10.3386/w25225.

Parigi, P., & Henson, W. (2014). Social isolation in America. *Annual Review of Sociology*, *40*(1), 153–171. https://doi.org/10.1146/annurev-soc-071312-145646.

Phelan, J. C., & Link, B. G. (2005). Controlling disease and creating disparities: A fundamental cause perspective. *The Journals of Gerontology: Series B*, *60*(Special_Issue_2), S27–S33. https://doi.org/10.1093/geronb/60.Special_Issue_2.S27.

Phelan, J. C., Link, B. G., & Tehranifar, P. (2010). Social conditions as fundamental causes of health inequalities: Theory, evidence, and policy implications. *Journal of Health and Social Behavior*, *51*(1_suppl), S28–S40. https://doi.org/10.1177/0022146510383498.

Pimouguet, C., Rizzuto, D., Schön, P., Shakersain, B., Angleman, S., Lagergren, M., Fratiglioni, L., & Xu, W. (2016). Impact of living alone on institutionalization and mortality: A population-based longitudinal study. *European Journal of Public Health*, *26*(1), 182–187. https://doi.org/10.1093/eurpub/ckv052.

Pollock, K. (2015). Is home always the best and preferred place of death? *British Medical Journal*, *351*. http://dx.doi.org/10.1136/bmj.h4855.

Putnam, R. D. (2001). *Bowling alone: The collapse and revival of American community*. Simon and Schuster.

Rogers, R. G. (1995). Marriage, sex, and mortality. *Journal of Marriage and Family*, *57*(2), 515–526. https://doi.org/10.2307/353703.

Rosso, A. L., Taylor, J. A., Tabb, L. P., & Michael, Y. L. (2013). Mobility, disability, and social engagement in older adults. *Journal of Aging and Health*, *25*(4), 617–637. https://doi.org/10.1177/0898264313482489.

Samuel, K., Alkire, S., Zavaleta, D., Mills, C., & Hammock, J. (2018). Social isolation and its relationship to multidimensional poverty. *Oxford Development Studies*, *46*(1), 83–97. https://doi.org/10.1080/13600818.2017.1311852.

Sand, L., & Strang, P. (2006). Existential loneliness in a palliative home care setting. *Journal of Palliative Medicine*, *9*(6), 1376–1387. https://doi.org/10.1089/jpm.2006.9.1376.

Sasson, I., & Umberson, D. J. (2014). Widowhood and depression: New light on gender differences, selection, and psychological adjustment. *The Journals of Gerontology: Series B*, *69B*(1), 135–145. https://doi.org/10.1093/geronb/gbt058.

Saver, J. L., Goyal, M., Lugt, A. van der, Menon, B. K., Majoie, C. B. L. M., Dippel, D. W., Campbell, B. C., Nogueira, R. G., Demchuk, A. M., Tomasello, A., Cardona, P., Devlin, T. G., Frei, D. F., Rochemont, R. du M. de, Berkhemer, O. A., Jovin, T. G., Siddiqui, A. H., Zwam, W. H. van, Davis, S. M., … Hill, M. D. (2016). Time to treatment with endovascular thrombectomy and outcomes from ischemic stroke: A meta-analysis. *Journal of the American Medical Association*, *316*(12), 1279–1289. https://doi.org/10.1001/jama.2016.13647.

Shankar, A., Hamer, M., McMunn, A., & Steptoe, A. (2013). Social isolation and loneliness: Relationships with cognitive function during 4 years of follow-up in the English Longitudinal Study of Ageing. *Psychosomatic Medicine, 75*(2), 161. https://doi.org/10.1097/PSY.0b013e31827f09cd.

Shankar, A., McMunn, A., Demakakos, P., Hamer, M., & Steptoe, A. (2017). Social isolation and loneliness: Prospective associations with functional status in older adults. *Health Psychology, 36*(2), 179–187. https://doi.org/10.1037/hea0000437.

Sherry, M., & Neller, A. (2016). Intellectual disability, stigma, and hate crimes. In K. Scior & S. Werner (Eds.), *Intellectual disability and stigma: Stepping out from the margins* (pp. 111–126). Palgrave Macmillan UK. https://doi.org/10.1057/978-1-137-52499-7_8.

Shye, D., Mullooly, J. P., Freeborn, D. K., & Pope, C. R. (1995). Gender differences in the relationship between social network support and mortality: A longitudinal study of an elderly cohort. *Social Science & Medicine, 41*(7), 935–947. https://doi.org/10.1016/0277-9536(94)00404-H.

Steptoe, A., Shankar, A., Demakakos, P., & Wardle, J. (2013). Social isolation, loneliness, and all-cause mortality in older men and women. *Proceedings of the National Academy of Sciences, 110*(15), 5797–5801. https://doi.org/10.1073/pnas.1219686110.

Thoits, P. A. (2011). Mechanisms linking social ties and support to physical and mental health. *Journal of Health and Social Behavior, 52*(2), 145–161. https://doi.org/10.1177/0022146510395592.

Todd, S. (2019, November 15). Why millennials never want to leave their apartment anymore. *Quartz*. https://qz.com/quartzy/1748191/how-millennials-became-a-generation-of-homebodies/.

U.S. Census Bureau. (2017). *Health insurance coverage in the United States: 2016*. www.census.gov/library/publications/2017/demo/p60-260.html.

Valtorta, N. K., Kanaan, M., Gilbody, S., Ronzi, S., & Hanratty, B. (2016). Loneliness and social isolation as risk factors for coronary heart disease and stroke: Systematic review and meta-analysis of longitudinal observational studies. *Heart, 102*(13), 1009–1016. https://doi.org/10.1136/heartjnl-2015-308790.

Weiss, B. D., Berman, E. A., Howe, C. L., & Fleming, R. B. (2012). Medical decision-making for older adults without family. *Journal of the American Geriatrics Society, 60*(11), 2144–2150. https://doi.org/10.1111/j.1532-5415.2012.04212.x.

Weiss, R. S. (1973). *Loneliness: The experience of emotional and social isolation*. The MIT Press.

Whittle, H. J., Palar, K., Ranadive, N. A., Turan, J. M., Kushel, M., & Weiser, S. D. (2017). "The land of the sick and the land of the healthy": Disability, bureaucracy, and stigma among people living with poverty and chronic illness in the United States. *Social Science & Medicine, 190*, 181–189. https://doi.org/10.1016/j.socscimed.2017.08.031.

Yuen, G. S., Bhutani, S., Lucas, B. J., Gunning, F. M., Abdel-Malak, B., Seirup, J. K., Klimstra, S. A., & Alexopoulos, G. S. (2015). Apathy in late-life depression: Common, persistent, and disabling. *The American Journal of Geriatric Psychiatry, 23*(5), 488–494. https://doi.org/10.1016/j.jagp.2014.06.005.

PART II
Public Issues

6
MEDICARE AND MEDICAID

This chapter covers the provisions of public policy that affect dying persons in the U.S. Despite having predictable death, the U.S. does not have explicit, comprehensive policy for the care of dying people. Rather, the same health care policies that affect people throughout the life course continue to apply to dying persons. Because most decedents are over the age of 65, Medicare policies are de facto end-of-life policies. Additionally, because most decedents require a period of long-term care before their deaths, Medicaid policies are also end-of-life policies. In this chapter, I describe relevant Medicare and Medicaid policies and the role the programs have played historically in reducing social disparities among older adults. I identify ways in which these policies affect hospice users as well as quality of care for very ill people who are not receiving hospice benefits. I address how end-of-life care affects health care costs nationwide. Finally, I explain the mechanisms for innovation built into Medicare and Medicaid.

The Role of Medicare and Medicaid in Addressing Social Disparities

Since 1965, older adults have had public health insurance through Medicare, and many long-term care recipients have had their costs covered through Medicaid. A person aged 65 or older can enroll in Medicare, provided that (a) he or she is a citizen or a legal permanent resident who has lived in the U.S. for at least five years, and (b) he or she has paid, or is married to someone who has paid, income taxes in the U.S. for ten years (Centers for Medicare & Medicaid Services, 2019a). Thus, Medicare is not strictly universal: Not all older people are eligible, and eligible older adults may choose to opt out of the program. But it is practically universal, such that in 2016, 1.2% of the population of adults aged 65 and older had no health insurance, 5.2% had private insurance only, and 93.6% had Medicare (U. S. Census Bureau, 2017). Medicare is not specifically a program for people who are dying; its services are available to enrollees regardless of prognosis. However, in 2014, 80% of people who died in the U.S. were people whose primary insurer was Medicare, so it is *effectively* the U.S. program for people who are dying (Cubanski et al., 2016). Therefore, Medicare policy defines end-of-life care (Huskamp et al., 2012).

About 20% of Medicare recipients are dual-eligible, meaning that they qualify for Medicaid, and therefore Medicare and Medicaid share the costs of their care (Henry J. Kaiser Family Foundation, 2018). Medicaid is intended for low-income, high-need Americans: minor children, their custodial parents, disabled persons, and persons requiring long-term care. Nationally, Medicaid covers approximately half of births, three-quarters of children in poverty, half of children and non-elderly adults with disabilities, and six in ten nursing home residents (Rudowitz et al., 2019). The modern long-term care industry would not exist without Medicaid, which paid $55 billion to nursing homes in 2015 alone (Henry J. Kaiser Family Foundation, 2017). Thus, Medicaid policy is de facto end-of-life policy primarily because one-third of people will need nursing home care at some point before their deaths (Henry J. Kaiser Family Foundation, 2017). After hospitals and private homes, nursing homes are the third most common places where deaths occur (Aldridge & Bradley, 2017). There is also a high rate of transitions in site of care in the last few months and even days of life, such that many deaths occur in hospitals or the homes of people who were recently under nursing home care (Aldridge & Bradley, 2017). Therefore, the design of Medicaid systems profoundly affects the care of dying people. For example, Medicaid reimbursement affects quality of care issues such as the number of nurses on staff (Harrington et al., 2006).

Medicare and Medicaid are some of the most successful social programs in the history of the United States, and they have changed the face of later life for millions of people. By the early 1960s – several years before Medicare and Medicaid became law in 1965 – conditions for older adults in the U.S. had become dire. Almost a third of older Americans lived below the poverty line, a higher percentage than any other age group (De Lew, 2000). Only 56% of people aged 65 and older had health insurance, because it was expensive and difficult to access (Moon, 1996). Until Congress passed the Affordable Care Act in 2010, private insurance companies could legally reject potential clients who might incur high costs, or disenroll current clients who were too expensive. Of course, older people were, and are, some of the most expensive patients, and private insurance companies would lose money insuring them. Additionally, most people in the U.S. accessed health insurance, as they do today, as a benefit of employment. Older adults who were too ill to work lost this access.

As a government program, Medicare took the responsibility of insuring older adults out of the private market. It had an immediate effect, with 19 million enrollees in 1966. Although the American Medical Association had bitterly opposed the law, 81% of physicians approved of it only 6 months after it was enacted (Colombotos, 1969). Use of care among Black and poor White older adults increased dramatically, and Medicare effectively ended racial segregation in hospitals (Donabedian, 1976; Gornick et al., 1996). By 1974, poverty rates among people 65 and older had dropped to 15%, and they have subsequently remained at or below the rates among younger persons (De Lew, 2000). Moreover, Medicare and Medicaid are more cost efficient than private health insurance (Wallace & Song, 2016). There is no doubt that without Medicare and Medicaid, far more older Americans and their families would be in poverty, and social disparities in health on the basis of age, race/ethnicity, and socioeconomic status would be much larger.

Thus, this chapter provides some responses to the effects of fundamental causes on inequalities in the predictable death. Fundamental causes call for "fundamental interventions" that act to interrupt social disparities in health by working to equalize opportunity (Reich et al., 2016, p. 185). National health policy is an area of fundamental intervention. Medicare alone is the nation's largest purchaser of health care services, giving it a great deal of power to alter systemic disparities (Eichner & Vladeck, 2005). Following countries such as the United Kingdom and New Zealand, some U.S. states are experimenting with tying Medicaid reimbursement to social determinants of health, due to evidence that delivering quality care is more expensive for people who face risks such as housing insecurity than for people who do not (Ash et al., 2017; Huffstetler & Phillips, 2019). Conversely, programs like Medicaid could use information about social risks in ways that inadvertently increase inequalities, such as imposing paid work requirements (Gottlieb & Alderwick, 2019).

The role of public policy in reducing inequalities in predictable death extends far beyond today's Medicare and Medicaid policies for current older adults. Medicaid, for example, covers children in poverty in part because intervention early in development, before the consequences of disadvantage have had time to accumulate, can yield health payoffs throughout the life course for future generations (Goldberg, 2014). Public health insurance options that extended throughout the life course, such as the proposed Medicare-for-all, would have the potential to eliminate inequalities that result from people being unable to afford health insurance in middle adulthood, when neither Medicare nor Medicaid offer coverage (Sohn, 2017).

Hospice Benefits

The programs have one benefit that is specifically for dying people. As described in Chapter 3, Medicare provides the hospice benefit for enrollees for whom a doctor has issued a prognosis of six months or less, and who agree to forgo Medicare payment for any subsequent curative treatment. Medicaid offers a nearly identical benefit because the two programs frequently share costs for dually eligible persons (Centers for Medicare & Medicaid Services, 2019b). The hospice benefit generally provides high value, with hospice patients receiving more comprehensive symptom control and less intensive medical intervention than dying patients who are not in hospice care (Higginson & Evans, 2010; Kelley et al., 2013). Thus I focus on problem areas in which redesign might better position hospice providers to meet the needs of dying persons, including updated reimbursement policies and better collaboration between Medicare and Medicaid.

Medicare reimburses hospices a per diem rate for each patient, and both the size of the reimbursement and its per diem structure pose some challenges to hospices. Until 2019, the reimbursement rate structure had changed little since the mid-1980s, when the benefit began (Centers for Medicare & Medicaid Services, 2019d; Huskamp et al., 2012). In 2019, Medicare responded to over a decade of government data indicating that the reimbursement rates did not reflect the actual costs of care. The law requires, however, that changes to hospice reimbursements be budget-neutral, meaning that increases in some reimbursements had to be offset with decreases in other reimbursements. The result was that Medicare increased the per diem reimbursements for care that takes place in hospitals, for respite care, and for 24-hour care at home. However, the per diem reimbursement for routine home care, which comprises 98% of hospice days, actually decreased (Centers for Medicare & Medicaid Services, 2019d).

Additionally, hospice is a volatile industry because its revenue stems from low Medicare reimbursement. Bankruptcy is a common problem (Ata et al., 2012) and profit margins are low (O'Neill et al., 2008). Over a ten-year period, 20% of hospices closed and another 40% changed owners (J. W. Thompson et al., 2012). Therefore, Medicare policies have an ultimate effect on whether patients have access to hospice care. These policies also structure the decisions of hospices, and thus the kinds of care that are available to patients. For example, reimbursement affects whether a hospice agency chooses to operate from within a nursing home or at patients' homes (Wiener & Tilly, 2003). It also structures business models: For-profit hospices have become increasingly common, with 80% of new hospice businesses being for-profit entities (J. W. Thompson et al., 2012).

In turn, a hospice's business model affects the kinds of patients it accepts and rejects. A per diem assumes that all patients cost about the same amount, or that low-cost patients will compensate for high-cost patients. In reality, the per diem rate means that hospices reject prospective patients whose palliation will be expensive (Aldridge et al., 2012; Huskamp et al., 2001). For-profit hospices, in particular, prefer patients whose primary need is assistance with daily living, such as dementia patients (Lorenz et al., 2004; Wachterman et al., 2011). The per diem policy also assumes that for a given patient, all days of care cost about the same amount, when in fact the beginning and end of hospice stays are significantly more expensive (Huskamp et al., 2008; Nicosia et al., 2009). Short hospice stays are therefore unprofitable for hospices, and so they reject prospective patients who may live only a few days (Lindrooth & Weisbrod, 2007; Noe & Forgione, 2014; Wachterman et al., 2011). Medicare adjusts its reimbursement rates for other benefits based on factors such as an organization's mix of clients, and such flexibility in the hospice benefit could help patients (Huskamp et al., 2012).

A second area in which the hospice might improve from redesign is the coordination of care for people who are dually eligible for both Medicare and Medicaid. In those cases, Medicare pays for the care itself, while Medicaid pays for the person's room and board in the facility where they are receiving long-term care (National Hospice and Palliative Care Organization, 2018). Medicaid has no incentive to reduce costs for Medicare, and vice versa. For example, Medicaid is unconcerned with the rates at which hospice patients are hospitalized, because Medicare pays for hospitalizations (Mor et al., 2010). This conflict produces quality of care issues for patients and their families.

Medicare and Medicaid Before Hospice

However, 52% of people who die are not receiving hospice care (National Hospice and Palliative Care Organization, 2017). Even hospice patients use other benefits in Medicare and Medicaid before they enter hospice. Thus, Medicare and Medicaid policies about services that the programs do and do not reimburse, and how much they pay for qualifying services, profoundly shape care for dying people well beyond the specific hospice benefit (DeWalt et al., 2005).

Medicare covers acute care needs such as short-term hospitalizations, surgeries, lab tests, outpatient visits, medical equipment, and prescription medications (Centers for Medicare & Medicaid Services, 2019c). It reimburses procedures, such as lab tests, much better than it reimburses practices such as history-taking, care coordination and management, and clinical assessment (Sinsky & Dugdale, 2013). Thus Medicare presents financial incentives for health care providers to spend the minimum amount of time on case management. Accordingly, two-thirds of decedents are hospitalized in the 6 months before death, and about one-fifth of deaths occur in hospitals (Dartmouth Institute for Health Policy and Clinical Practice, 2019).

For older adults, Medicaid covers long-term care when patients are out of money to do so themselves. Older adults usually pay for long-term care out of pocket until they have spent down their assets so as to be eligible for Medicaid. The average annual cost of a nursing home in 2016 was $82,000, and so most people come to the end of their means rather quickly (Henry J. Kaiser Family Foundation, 2017). Medicaid reimburses long-term care providers less than the full cost of the services they provide (S. Zuckerman et al., 2009). Therefore, some nursing homes reject Medicaid patients (Decker, 2012).

Beyond these broad incentives, Medicare and Medicaid policies affect the end-of-life care that people receive in specific ways. To demonstrate, I cover the case of post-acute care quality in Medicare and the case of long-term care quality in Medicaid. Post-acute care is rehabilitative and continuing care that occurs after an emergency, but before the patient is either entirely well or stable enough to move to long-term care (Medpac, 2019). Medicare pays for a short period of post-acute care, and increasing use and intensity of this care has become an important driver of growth in Medicare spending (Chandra et al., 2013). Therefore, Medicare is interested in curbing unnecessary post-acute care, but it is also interested in reducing the rate of rehospitalizations and the number of overall transitions in site of care. Transitions are expensive, they are common, they compromise care quality and patient safety, and they are preventable (Coleman et al., 2004; Mor et al., 2010). Among dying persons, the average patient experiences three transitions in the last three months of life (Teno et al., 2013).

Decisions about receipt of acute care, post-acute care, and transitions between the two should, in theory, be based on a physician's assessment of the patient's condition. However, many studies indicate that Medicare reimbursement, and changes in Medicare reimbursement structure, are in fact the major determinants of physicians' decisions. These include decisions about the setting for post-acute care, such as at home versus in a skilled nursing facility (Buntin et al., 2009; Grabowski et al., 2012) and time of discharge from post-acute care (Kim et al., 2015).

Medicaid goes on to shape the care people receive when they transition from post-acute care to long-term care. The Centers for Medicare and Medicaid Services (CMS), an agency within the federal government, regulates quality standards in nursing homes and other long-term care settings that receive reimbursement from Medicaid. (For a brief history of nursing home quality standards, see Castle & Ferguson, 2010.) When a patient is initially admitted to a nursing home, the staff completes a form called the Resident Assessment Instrument (RAI). The RAI, sometimes also known as a Resident Assessment Protocol, is a statement about the patient's current condition that further includes evaluation and planning features. The nursing home, patient, and family identify desired outcomes for the patient and establish a plan of action to achieve them (Centers for Medicare & Medicaid Services, 2017a). CMS requires RAI information for every patient in a facility, regardless of whether the patient is receiving Medicare or Medicaid. Each patient's RAI is updated every three months, as well as when the patient experiences a major health event.

The nursing home forwards RAI information to the state, and the state forwards this information to the national CMS database, which is called the Minimum Data Set (Centers for Medicare & Medicaid Services, 2017b). This information is available to the public for consumers to access when they are choosing a nursing home. The Minimum Data Set also permits nursing homes to compare and contrast themselves with other facilities, and permits the government to identify areas in which nursing homes as a class are excelling or lacking. Finally, individual nursing homes with significant problems face sanctions, ranging from monetary fines to enhanced state monitoring to being disqualified from receiving reimbursement from Medicare and Medicaid.

The information required on the RAI, then, shapes the practices of nursing homes: They focus on features included on the RAI and spend less time and energy on aspects of care that are not documented on the RAI. For example, critics note that many nursing homes neglect quality of *life*, because the RAI emphasizes quality of *care* (Kane, 2003). That is, nursing homes are required to report the proportion of residents with whom they are employing physical or medicinal restraints, but they do not report the proportion of residents who rate quality of life at the facility to be excellent. A related concern is that the RAI system may cause nursing homes to spend their time in narrow-scope striving to score well on the indicators, rather than striving more broadly to provide high-quality care (Rahman & Applebaum, 2009). Expert clinicians conclude that the RAI only approximates guidelines for best clinical practice (Dosa et al., 2006). Of course, the system undergoes revisions over time, with a major 2010 revision increasing the emphasis facilities place on residents' own opinions and reports, such as preferences for care (Saliba et al., 2012). However, revisions are generally in response to critiques, rather than in anticipation of potential problems.

The RAI is in some ways inconsistent with quality of care for dying persons. RAI care plans are designed to focus on restoration of prior function and/or maintenance of current function. Dying people inevitably experience declines, even under aggressive rehabilitative care. For example, weight loss is an indicator of problems on the RAI, but it is normal in dying patients (Wiener & Tilly, 2003). The law was amended in 1989 to allow hospice care in RAI plans, but plans still tend to emphasize rehabilitation over palliation (S. Thompson & Oliver, 2008). Therefore, symptoms such as untreated pain remain a problem for people dying in nursing homes (Buchanan et al., 2002). Research and pilot testing is ongoing for RAIs that are tailored to hospice patients (Hermans et al., 2018; Mukamel et al., 2016).

The Role of Death and Dying in Overall Healthcare Costs

People care about the high cost of medical care because everyone pays for it: The cost of care comes either directly from people's pockets, or indirectly from them via taxes and other public funds. On the surface, end-of-life care appears to be extremely expensive. In 2014, Medicare spent an average of $34,529 on each person who died, compared with $9,121 on each person who survived the year (Cubanski et al., 2016). Inpatient hospital care accounted for most of the difference. Therefore, an easy assumption is that there is profligate spending on hospital-based life-saving measures that fail.

However, that perception is not accurate. Only 12% of people who die incur high costs that are limited to the final 12 months of their lives (Davis et al., 2016; French et al., 2017). Rather, there is a small group of patients who incur extremely high costs for years before they die: 5% of the population accounts for 49% of annual health care spending (Stanton & Rutherford, 2005). Such people are often disabled adults in middle and later life who have multiple chronic illnesses that require complex care and careful case management (Sommers & Cohen, 2006). These high-cost patients comprise a large proportion of the people who die each year, but most high-cost patients survive more than 1 year (Aldridge & Kelley, 2015). In other words, the problem is not a sudden spike in medical intervention at the end of life, but rather a group of very ill people for whom health care costs are persistently high until they die (Einav et al., 2018).

Thus, wider use of hospice has the potential to reduce overall health care costs, but reducing costs in the last six months of life only solves part of the problem. Further, although hospice is often lower-tech than standard treatment, it is not always correspondingly less expensive. Some studies conclude that hospice is more expensive in the last months of life than standard treatment (Gozalo et al., 2015), while others conclude that it is less expensive (Kelley et al., 2013; Obermeyer et al., 2014). To some extent, the difference in results is due to research methods, with scholars noting that results depend on the amount of time before death that is examined and whether a study is cross-sectional or longitudinal (Unroe et al., 2016). However, there are also real nuances to the issue. One is that hospice is less expensive than standard care for some patients, but not others. For example, it saves money for lung cancer patients who are dying in nursing homes, but not among Alzheimer's patients who are not institutionalized (R. B. Zuckerman et al., 2016). Another nuance is that hospice may save money in regions of the country that have high average health care costs, but not in regions of the country that already have low costs (Wang et al., 2017). A third nuance is that duration of hospice care matters, with many patients referred too late for hospice to affect costs at all (Wachterman et al., 2018). Thus, there is potential for Medicare and Medicaid to better structure the benefit to capitalize on cost savings while making hospice more consistently accessible to a wider variety of patients.

Because the high costs of care for critically ill people extend more than six months before death, cost savings must result from changes to general Medicare and Medicaid policy in addition to the specific hospice benefit. There are a variety of approaches along these lines, intended to reduce costs for the small proportion of patients whose care is exceedingly expensive yet who may survive several more years. First, palliative care experts are interested in expanding the use of symptom management and care coordination to people who do not qualify for the hospice benefit (Meier et al., 2017). These experts suppose that palliative care reduces the cost of care, which is an open question. Very little is known about the cost of palliative care among people who are not hospice-eligible, because insurance rules render palliative care prohibitively expensive for most people.

A second group of experts interested in cost reductions is focused on creating econometric models that prospectively identify patients who are at risk of incurring high costs in the future. The hope is that prevention could reduce later costly care needs more effectively than intervention that begins only after people have already become high-cost care users. For example, people with multiple chronic illnesses, people who have a history of substance abuse, people living with housing and food insecurity, and people with mental illnesses tend to become high-cost care users (Billings & Mijanovich, 2007; de Oliveira et al., 2016; Fitzpatrick et al., 2015). Much of this work aims to improve the forecasting models that Medicare and Medicaid might adopt (Chechulin et al., 2014; Meenan et al., 1999). Another angle on the issue is to aim to identify not only which patients could become high cost, but also which of those patients' cases might be most amenable to intervention (Lewis, 2010).

Finally, a third group of experts has designed Medicare and Medicaid interventions for high-cost patients and for individuals at risk of becoming high-cost patients. For example, in New Jersey, health care providers who accept Medicaid can form accountable care organizations (ACOs) focusing on high-cost patients in high-poverty areas of the state (Cantor et al., 2014). An innovation of the 2010 Affordable Care Act, ACOs are a mechanism to use public money to reward health care providers for what they do to keep patients healthy, rather than to reimburse them for treatment delivered. The research evaluating interventions such as this has made clear that no single type of intervention will solve the problem. For example, many had high hopes for improved case management as a strategy to reduce costs and improve outcomes. The thinking was that if a case manager could coordinate various specialists as well as assess the patient's social service needs, care would become more streamlined and efficient, and thereby cost less. Unfortunately, a meta-analysis of 36 case management interventions showed no significant overall cost savings (Stokes et al., 2015). Case management interventions need to be very carefully designed to work. Certain elements, such as in-person contact rather than digital medicine, and interdisciplinary management teams rather than individual case managers, appear to be most successful (Lee et al., 2018).

A final complexity is designing a set of policies that maximally enhance access to and quality of care while simultaneously maintaining or lowering cost (Schoen et al., 2010). An efficient system in which money is only spend on effective care is not easy to achieve (Orszag & Emanuel, 2010). For example, an article in the *New England Journal of Medicine* rated health care systems on the cost of their services relative to the amount of high-quality extended life that people receive from the services (Weinstein & Skinner, 2010). They found that there is not a simple correlation between health care spending and patient outcomes. A system that waits until heart disease patients become very ill and then treats them intensively, for example, will worsen patient outcomes if all it does is reduce intensive interventions. It also must increase spending on more efficient treatments, such as prevention with aspirin or beta-blockers. Thus paradoxically, health care systems are often inefficient because of the efficient care they are *not* providing, rather than solely because of the high cost of the inefficient care they are providing.

Moreover, the decisions an efficient system makes can be unpopular and seem unfeeling at the level of individual patients. For example, the United Kingdom has a public health care system that deliberately makes it difficult to get very expensive cancer treatments that are unlikely to lengthen patients' lives by more than a few days or weeks. Yet when individual patients request exceptions, even panels of neutral experts have great difficulty deciding who should receive them (Hughes & Doheny, 2019a, 2019b).

Mechanisms for Innovation in Medicare and Medicaid

Since 1983, a waivers program has operated within Medicare and Medicaid to encourage pilot or demonstration projects that may lead to larger reforms of the programs (Centers for Medicare and Medicaid Services, 2018). Increasingly, new waivers address the needs of dually eligible patients. Initially, a waiver covers five years, and can be renewed every three years indefinitely. Thus there are multiple, long-standing waivers in most states, and a small number of programs that began as waivers programs have been legislated permanently into Medicare or Medicaid.

The federal government requires state Medicaid programs to pay only for long-term care in institutions such as nursing homes. Almost all home and community-based services, which allow organizations to administer care outside of an institutional setting while still receiving Medicaid reimbursement, operate through a waivers program (Centers for Medicare and Medicaid Services, 2018). Home and community-based services are extremely popular, such that in 2016, 57% of Medicaid spending on long-term care went to home and community-based services rather than to institutional care (Watts et al., 2020). These waivers programs add a flexibility to Medicaid that meets client demand while also satisfying budget officials. Most older adults who have long-term care needs strongly prefer to remain at home rather than moving to an institutional setting, and they wish to die at home as well when the time comes (Gomes et al., 2013). Moreover, home and community-based services may be less expensive than institution-based services, allowing states to save money (Kitchener et al., 2006; Wysocki et al., 2012). The Supreme Court's *Olmstead* decision in 1999 helped solidify the existence of home and community-based services: The Court ruled that it is illegal discrimination to institutionalize people with disabilities who could, with proper support, live in the community (Musumeci & Claypool, 2014).

However, most home and community-based services programs remain waivers programs, which involves several significant drawbacks. First, waivers programs are optional for states to offer, and thus not guaranteed to be available in the future. Medicaid is currently an entitlement program, meaning that the federal government matches state spending regardless of how high that spending may go. The Trump administration would prefer to limit federal health care spending by issuing each state a fixed block grant, rather than a blank check, to operate Medicaid (Sachs & Huberfeld, 2019). That kind of reform would in turn greatly limit which services a state could afford to offer its residents, such that non-mandatory programs such as waivers could be reduced significantly.

A second significant drawback to waivers programs is that unlike federally required aspects of Medicaid, states may set limits on how many people can receive their services through a waivers program. As a result, in 2017, there were 700,000 people across the nation on waiting lists for home and community-based services, and that number has increased by an average of 9% each year since 2000 (Musumeci et al., 2019). Some of these people will die in institutions, or without services, in the average of 30 months before they can get off the waiting list and into the program (Musumeci et al., 2019).

Programs that leave waivers status to become legislated permanently into Medicare or Medicaid are on much stronger footing. One such permanent alternative to nursing home care is the Program of All-Inclusive Care for the Elderly (PACE). The On Lok Senior Services program, designed in the early 1970s to provide services to frail older adults in San Francisco's Chinatown, is the basis for PACE. With waivers and additional grant assistance from the Robert Wood Johnson Foundation, the program spread and expanded until it became a formal option within Medicare in 1997 (Centers for Medicare and Medicaid Services, 2011). The goal of PACE is to provide whatever services are necessary to help older adults who need nursing home levels of care to continue living outside of nursing homes (National PACE Association, 2016). Medicare and Medicaid pay a single organization, PACE, to coordinate each patient's care under an interdisciplinary team of health care professionals, social workers, and others. Thus PACE is all-inclusive of medical needs including preventive, acute, post-acute, and long-term care, and also of social needs such as transportation and nutrition that might otherwise require a person to move to a nursing home. In 2018 there were 124 organizations in 31 states that were operating a PACE (National PACE Association, 2018). Most PACE providers are non-profit businesses, although for-profit PACE models exist as well (Centers for Medicare & Medicaid Services, 2015).

PACE is not specifically a program for dying persons, but it does provide comprehensive care for patients who are dying. PACE programs have very high rates of advance care planning among their participants (Pak et al., 2012; Schamp & Tenkku, 2006). Because of their contact with the same patients over time, even unskilled members of the interdisciplinary teams are able to identify when patients have reached the end of life and need to alter care plans accordingly (Meeker & Waldrop, 2017). PACE has proven to be a good model for delivering end-of-life care that is consistent with patients' preferences, and for reducing hospitalization at the end of life (Schamp & Tenkku, 2006; Segelman et al., 2014; Temkin-Greener & Mukamel, 2002). Because it is not subject to usual Medicare and Medicaid rules, it can offer palliative care to people who do not have a six-month prognosis and who do not wish to give up other treatment (Eng, 2002). Thus end-of-life care through PACE can be more consistent and integrated than hospice. A limitation that PACE professionals report is that sometimes they are unable to provide appropriate end-of-life services in the community setting, such that a nursing home would better suit some patients' needs (Meeker & Waldrop, 2017). In some locations, PACE and hospice have entered into collaborations (National Hospice and Palliative Care Organization, 2012).

Summary

Eight in ten of the people who die each year are insured through Medicare; of those, a proportion is dually eligible for Medicaid. Medicaid funds six in ten nursing home stays. Therefore, Medicare and Medicaid policies greatly influence end-of-life care in the U.S. The hospice benefit provides palliative care to people who have a prognosis of six months or less to live and who agree to stop any care designed to cure them. Beyond this specific end-of-life provision that is common to both programs, there are few specific policies for dying persons. Nevertheless, Medicare and Medicaid rules affect the quality of care that dying people receive, the reimbursement incentives that health care professionals use to prescribe care, and the costs that both individual families and taxpayers pay for care for dying people. The programs experiment with innovations aimed at improving quality of care and cost issues, and pilot initiatives that work, such as the Program of All-Inclusive Care for the Elderly, have become permanent parts of Medicare and Medicaid law. Overall, Medicare and Medicaid are vital public programs to older adults, both before and throughout the dying process.

References

Aldridge, M. D., Barry, C. L., Cherlin, E. J., McCorkle, R., & Bradley, E. H. (2012). Hospices' enrollment policies may contribute to underuse of hospice care in the United States. *Health Affairs, 31*(12), 2690–2698. https://doi.org/10.1377/hlthaff.2012.0286.

Aldridge, M. D., & Bradley, E. H. (2017). Epidemiology and patterns of care at the end of life: Rising complexity, shifts in care patterns and sites of death. *Health Affairs, 36*(7), 1175–1183. https://doi.org/10.1377/hlthaff.2017.0182.

Aldridge, M. D., & Kelley, A. S. (2015). The myth regarding the high cost of end-of-life care. *American Journal of Public Health, 105*(12), 2411–2415. https://doi.org/10.2105/AJPH.2015.302889.

Ash, A. S., Mick, E. O., Ellis, R. P., Kiefe, C. I., Allison, J. J., & Clark, M. A. (2017). Social determinants of health in managed care payment formulas. *JAMA Internal Medicine, 177*(10), 1424–1430. https://doi.org/10.1001/jamainternmed.2017.3317.

Ata, B., Killaly, B. L., Olsen, T. L., & Parker, R. P. (2012). On hospice operations under Medicare reimbursement policies. *Management Science, 59*(5), 1027–1044. https://doi.org/10.1287/mnsc.1120.1606.

Billings, J., & Mijanovich, T. (2007). Improving the management of care for high-cost Medicaid patients. *Health Affairs, 26*(6), 1643–1654. https://doi.org/10.1377/hlthaff.26.6.1643.

Buchanan, R. J., Choi, M., Wang, S., & Huang, C. (2002). Analyses of nursing home residents in hospice care using the Minimum Data Set. *Palliative Medicine, 16*(6), 465–480. https://doi.org/10.1191/0269216302pm589oa.

Buntin, M. B., Colla, C. H., & Escarce, J. J. (2009). Effects of payment changes on trends in post-acute care. *Health Services Research, 44*(4), 1188–1210. https://doi.org/10.1111/j.1475-6773.2009.00968.x.

Cantor, J. C., Chakravarty, S., Tong, J., Yedidia, M. J., Lontok, O., & DeLia, D. (2014). The New Jersey Medicaid ACO demonstration project: Seeking opportunities for better care and lower costs among complex low-income patients. *Journal of Health Politics, Policy and Law, 39*(6), 1185–1211. https://doi.org/10.1215/03616878-2822622.

Castle, N. G., & Ferguson, J. C. (2010). What is nursing home quality and how is it measured? *The Gerontologist, 50*(4), 426–442. https://doi.org/10.1093/geront/gnq052.

Centers for Medicare & Medicaid Services. (2015). *Private, for-profit demo project for the Program of All-Inclusive Care for the Elderly (PACE).* https://innovation.cms.gov/initiatives/PACE/.

Centers for Medicare & Medicaid Services. (2017a). *Long-term care facility resident assessment instrument 3.0 user's manual.* https://downloads.cms.gov/files/1-MDS-30-RAI-Manual-v115R-October-1-2017-R.pdf.

Centers for Medicare & Medicaid Services. (2017b). *Nursing home quality initiative.* www.cms.gov/Medicare/Quality-Initiatives-Patient-Assessment-Instruments/NursingHomeQualityInits/index.html.

Centers for Medicare & Medicaid Services. (2019a). *Eligibility & premium calculator.* www.medicare.gov/eligibilitypremiumcalc/.

Centers for Medicare & Medicaid Services. (2019b). *Hospice benefits.* www.medicaid.gov/medicaid/benefits/hospice/index.html.

Centers for Medicare & Medicaid Services. (2019c). *What Medicare covers.* www.medicare.gov/what-medicare-covers/.

Centers for Medicare & Medicaid Services. (2019d). *Medicare program; FY 2020 hospice wage index and payment rate update and hospice quality reporting requirements* (No. 2019–16583). www.federalregister.gov/documents/2019/08/06/2019-16583/medicare-program-fy-2020-hospice-wage-index-and-payment-rate-update-and-hospice-quality-reporting.

Centers for Medicare and Medicaid Services. (2011). *Programs of All-Inclusive Care for the Elderly (PACE).* www.cms.gov/Regulations-and-Guidance/Guidance/Manuals/downloads/pace111c01.pdf.

Centers for Medicare and Medicaid Services. (2018). *National overview of 1915(c) HCBS waivers.* www.cms.gov/Outreach-and-Education/American-Indian-Alaska-Native/AIAN/LTSS-TA-Center/info/national-overview-1915-c-waivers.html.

Chandra, A., Dalton, M. A., & Holmes, J. (2013). Large increases in spending on postacute care in Medicare point to the potential for cost savings in these settings. *Health Affairs, 32*(5), 864–872. https://doi.org/10.1377/hlthaff.2012.1262.

Chechulin, Y., Nazerian, A., Rais, S., & Malikov, K. (2014). Predicting patients with high risk of becoming high-cost healthcare users in Ontario (Canada). *Healthcare Policy, 9*(3), 68–79.

Coleman, E. A., Min, S., Chomiak, A., & Kramer, A. M. (2004). Posthospital care transitions: Patterns, complications, and risk identification. *Health Services Research, 39*(5), 1449–1466. https://doi.org/10.1111/j.1475-6773.2004.00298.x.

Colombotos, J. (1969). Physicians and Medicare: A before-after study of the effects of legislation on attitudes. *American Sociological Review, 34*(3), 318–334. https://doi.org/10.2307/2092498.

Cubanski, J., Neuman, T., Griffin, S., & Damico, A. (2016). *Medicare spending at the end of life: A snapshot of beneficiaries who died in 2014 and the cost of their care.* Henry J. Kaiser Family Foundation. www.kff.org/medicare/issue-brief/medicare-spending-at-the-end-of-life/.

Dartmouth Institute for Health Policy and Clinical Practice. (2019). *Dartmouth atlas of health care*. www.dartmouthatlas.org/data/table.aspx?ind=15.

Davis, M. A., Nallamothu, B. K., Banerjee, M., & Bynum, J. P.W. (2016). Identification of four unique spending patterns among older adults in the last year of life challenges standard assumptions. *Health Affairs, 35*(7), 1316–1323. https://doi.org/10.1377/hlthaff.2015.1419.

De Lew, N. (2000). Medicare: 35 years of service. *Health Care Financing Review, 22*(1), 75–103.

de Oliveira, C., Cheng, J., Vigod, S., Rehm, J., & Kurdyak, P. (2016). Patients with high mental health costs incur over 30 percent more costs than other high-cost patients. *Health Affairs, 35*(1), 36–43. https://doi.org/10.1377/hlthaff.2015.0278.

Decker, S. L. (2012). In 2011 nearly one-third of physicians said they would not accept new Medicaid patients, but rising fees may help. *Health Affairs, 31*(8), 1673–1679. https://doi.org/10.1377/hlthaff.2012.0294.

DeWalt, D. A., Oberlander, J., Carey, T. S., & Roper, W. L. (2005). Significance of Medicare and Medicaid programs for the practice of medicine. *Health Care Financing Review, 27*(2), 79–90.

Donabedian, A. (1976). Effects of Medicare and Medicaid on access to and quality of health care. *Public Health Reports, 91*(4), 322–331.

Dosa, D., Bowers, B., & Gifford, D. R. (2006). Critical review of resident assessment protocols. *Journal of the American Geriatrics Society, 54*(4), 659–666. https://doi.org/10.1111/j.1532-5415.2006.00654.x.

Eichner, J., & Vladeck, B. C. (2005). Medicare as a catalyst for reducing health disparities. *Health Affairs, 24*(2), 365–375. https://doi.org/10.1377/hlthaff.24.2.365.

Einav, L., Finkelstein, A., Mullainathan, S., & Obermeyer, Z. (2018). Predictive modeling of U.S. health care spending in late life. *Science, 360*(6396), 1462–1465. https://doi.org/10.1126/science.aar5045.

Eng, C. (2002). Future consideration for improving end-of-life care for older persons: Program of All-inclusive Care for the Elderly (PACE). *Journal of Palliative Medicine, 5*(2), 305–310. https://doi.org/10.1089/109662102753641313.

Fitzpatrick, T., Rosella, L. C., Calzavara, A., Petch, J., Pinto, A. D., Manson, H., Goel, V., & Wodchis, W. P. (2015). Looking beyond income and education: Socioeconomic status gradients among future high-cost users of health care. *American Journal of Preventive Medicine, 49*(2), 161–171. https://doi.org/10.1016/j.amepre.2015.02.018.

French, E. B., McCauley, J., Aragon, M., Bakx, P., Chalkley, M., Chen, S. H., Christensen, B. J., Chuang, H., Côté-Sergent, A., De Nardi, M., Fan, E., Échevin, D., Geoffard, P.-Y., Gastaldi-Ménager, C., Gørtz, M., Ibuka, Y., Jones, J. B., Kallestrup-Lamb, M., Karlsson, M., … Kelly, E. (2017). End-of-life medical spending in last twelve months of life is lower than previously reported. *Health Affairs, 36*(7), 1211–1217. https://doi.org/10.1377/hlthaff.2017.0174.

Goldberg, D. S. (2014). The implications of fundamental cause theory for priority setting. *American Journal of Public Health, 104*(10), 1839–1843. https://doi.org/10.2105/AJPH.2014.302058.

Gomes, B., Calanzani, N., Gysels, M., Hall, S., & Higginson, I. J. (2013). Heterogeneity and changes in preferences for dying at home: A systematic review. *BMC Palliative Care, 12*(1), 7. https://doi.org/10.1186/1472-684X-12-7.

Gornick, M. E., Warren, J. L., Eggers, P. W., Lubitz, J. D., De Lew, N., Davis, M. H., & Cooper, B. S. (1996). Thirty years of Medicare: Impact on the covered population. *Health Care Financing Review, 18*(2), 179–237.

Gottlieb, L. M., & Alderwick, H. (2019). Integrating social and medical care: Could it worsen health and increase inequity? *The Annals of Family Medicine, 17*(1), 77–81. https://doi.org/10.1370/afm.2339.

Gozalo, P., Plotzke, M., Mor, V., Miller, S. C., & Teno, J. M. (2015). Changes in Medicare costs with the growth of hospice care in nursing homes. *New England Journal of Medicine, 372*(19), 1823–1831. https://doi.org/10.1056/NEJMsa1408705.

Grabowski, D. C., Huckfeldt, P. J., Sood, N., Escarce, J. J., & Newhouse, J. P. (2012). Medicare postacute care payment reforms have potential to improve efficiency of care, but may need changes to cut costs. *Health Affairs, 31*(9), 1941–1950. https://doi.org/10.1377/hlthaff.2012.0351.

Harrington, C., Swan, J. H., & Carrillo, H. (2006). Nurse staffing levels and Medicaid reimbursement rates in nursing facilities. *Health Services Research, 42*, 1105–1129. https://doi.org/10.1111/j.1475-6773.2006.00641.x.

Henry J. Kaiser Family Foundation. (2017). *Medicaid's role in nursing home care*. www.kff.org/infographic/medicaids-role-in-nursing-home-care/.

Henry J. Kaiser Family Foundation. (2018). *Dual eligibles as a percent of total Medicare beneficiaries*. www.kff.org/medicaid/state-indicator/duals-as-a-of-medicare-beneficiaries/.

Hermans, K., Mello, J. D. A., Spruytte, N., Cohen, J., Audenhove, C. V., & Declercq, A. (2018). Does using the interRAI Palliative Care instrument reduce the needs and symptoms of nursing home residents receiving palliative care? *Palliative & Supportive Care, 16*(1), 32–40. https://doi.org/10.1017/S1478951517000153.

Higginson, I. J., & Evans, C. J. (2010). What is the evidence that palliative care teams improve outcomes for cancer patients and their families? *The Cancer Journal, 16*(5), 423. https://doi.org/10.1097/PPO.0b013e3181f684e5.

Huffstetler, A. N., & Phillips, R. L. (2019). Payment structures that support social care integration with clinical care: Social deprivation indices and novel payment models. *American Journal of Preventive Medicine, 57*(6, Supplement 1), S82–S88. https://doi.org/10.1016/j.amepre.2019.07.011.

Hughes, D., & Doheny, S. (2019a). Constructing 'exceptionality': A neglected aspect of NHS rationing. *Sociology of Health & Illness, 41*(8), 1600–1617. https://doi.org/10.1111/1467-9566.12976.

Hughes, D., & Doheny, S. (2019b). Doing evidence-based medicine? How NHS managers ration high-cost drugs. *Social Science & Medicine, 235*(C), 1–1.

Huskamp, H. A., Buntin, M. B., Wang, V., & Newhouse, J. P. (2001). Providing care at the end of life: Do Medicare rules impede good care? *Health Affairs, 20*(3), 204–211. https://doi.org/10.1377/hlthaff.20.3.204.

Huskamp, H. A., Kaufmann, C., & Stevenson, D. G. (2012). The intersection of long-term care and end-of-life care. *Medical Care Research and Review, 69*(1), 3–44. https://doi.org/10.1177/1077558711418518.

Huskamp, H. A., Newhouse, J. P., Norcini, J. C., & Keating, N. L. (2008). Variation in patients' hospice costs. *INQUIRY: The Journal of Health Care Organization, Provision, and Financing, 45*(2), 232–244. https://doi.org/10.5034/inquiryjrnl_45.02.232.

Kane, R. A. (2003). Definition, measurement, and correlates of quality of life in nursing homes: Toward a reasonable practice, research, and policy agenda. *The Gerontologist, 43*(suppl_2), 28–36. https://doi.org/10.1093/geront/43.suppl_2.28.

Kelley, A. S., Deb, P., Du, Q., Aldridge Carlson, M. D., & Morrison, R. S. (2013). Hospice enrollment saves money for Medicare and improves care quality across a number of different lengths-of-stay. *Health Affairs, 32*(3), 552–561. https://doi.org/10.1377/hlthaff.2012.0851.

Kim, Y. S., Kleerup, E. C., Ganz, P. A., Ponce, N. A., Lorenz, K. A., & Needleman, J. (2015). Medicare payment policy creates incentives for long-term care hospitals to time discharges for maximum reimbursement. *Health Affairs, 34*(6), 907–915. https://doi.org/10.1377/hlthaff.2014.0778.

Kitchener, M., Ng, T., Miller, N., & Harrington, C. (2006). Institutional and community-based long-term care. *Journal of Health & Social Policy, 22*(2), 31–50. https://doi.org/10.1300/J045v22n02_03.

Lee, J. Y., Muratov, S., Tarride, J.-E., & Holbrook, A. M. (2018). Managing high-cost healthcare users: The international search for effective evidence-supported strategies. *Journal of the American Geriatrics Society, 66*(5), 1002–1008. https://doi.org/10.1111/jgs.15257.

Lewis, G. H. (2010). "Impactibility models:" Identifying the subgroup of high-risk patients most amenable to hospital-avoidance programs. *The Milbank Quarterly, 88*(2), 240–255. https://doi.org/10.1111/j.1468-0009.2010.00597.x.

Lindrooth, R. C., & Weisbrod, B. A. (2007). Do religious nonprofit and for-profit organizations respond differently to financial incentives? The hospice industry. *Journal of Health Economics, 26*(2), 342–357. https://doi.org/10.1016/j.jhealeco.2006.09.003.

Lorenz, K. A., Asch, S. M., Rosenfeld, K. E., Liu, H., & Ettner, S. L. (2004). Hospice admission practices: Where does hospice fit in the continuum of care? *Journal of the American Geriatrics Society, 52*(5), 725–730. https://doi.org/10.1111/j.1532-5415.2004.52209.x.

Medpac. (2019). *Post-acute care*. www.medpac.gov/-research-areas-/post-acute-care.

Meeker, M. A., & Waldrop, D. P. (2017). Changing focus: End-of-life care in a New York State managed long-term care program. *Journal of Applied Gerontology*, 073346481773762. https://doi.org/10.1177/0733464817737620.

Meenan, R. T., O'Keeffe-Rosetti, M. C., Hornbrook, M. C., Bachman, D. J., Goodman, M. J., Fishman, P. A., & Hurtado, A. V. (1999). The sensitivity and specificity of forecasting high-cost users of medical care. *Medical Care, 37*(8), 815. https://doi.org/10.1097/00005650-199908000-00011.

Meier, D. E., Back, A. L., Berman, A., Block, S. D., Corrigan, J. M., & Morrison, R. S. (2017). A national strategy for palliative care. *Health Affairs, 36*(7), 1265–1273. https://doi.org/10.1377/hlthaff.2017.0164.

Moon, M. (1996). What Medicare has meant to older Americans. *Health Care Financing Review, 18*(2), 49–59.

Mor, V., Intrator, O., Feng, Z., & Grabowski, D. C. (2010). The revolving door of rehospitalization from skilled nursing facilities. *Health Affairs, 29*(1), 57–64. https://doi.org/10.1377/hlthaff.2009.0629.

Mukamel, D. B., Ladd, H., Caprio, T., & Temkin-Greener, H. (2016). Prototype end-of-life quality measures based on MDS 3 data. *Medical Care, 54*(11), 1024. https://doi.org/10.1097/MLR.0000000000000576.

Musumeci, M., Chidambaram, P., & Watts, M. O. (2019). *Key questions about Medicaid home and community-based services waiver waiting lists*. Kaiser Family Foundation. www.kff.org/medicaid/issue-brief/key-questions-about-medicaid-home-and-community-based-services-waiver-waiting-lists/.

Musumeci, M., & Claypool, H. (2014). *Olmstead's role in community integration for people with disabilities under medicaid: 15 years after the Supreme Court's Olmstead decision*. Kaiser Family Foundation. www.kff.org/medicaid/issue-brief/olmsteads-role-in-community-integration-for-people-with-disabilities-under-medicaid-15-years-after-the-supreme-courts-olmstead-decision/.

National Hospice and Palliative Care Organization. (2012). *NHPCO facts and figures on hospice care in America.* www.nhpco.org/sites/default/files/public/newsline/2012/NL_March_12.pdf.

National Hospice and Palliative Care Organization. (2017). *Facts and figures: Hospice care in America.* www.nhpco.org/sites/default/files/public/Statistics_Research/2017_Facts_Figures.pdf.

National Hospice and Palliative Care Organization. (2018). *Medicaid issue brief.* www.nhpco.org/sites/default/files/public/regulatory/Medicaid_Issue_Brief.pdf.

National PACE Association. (2016). *Understanding PACE.* www.npaonline.org/sites/default/files/Profile%20of%20PACE_December%202016.pdf.

National PACE Association. (2018). *PACE in the states.* www.npaonline.org/sites/default/files/PDFs/PACE%20in%20the%20States%20June%202018.pdf.

Nicosia, N., Reardon, E., Lorenz, K., Lynn, J., & Buntin, M. B. (2009). The Medicare hospice payment system: A consideration of potential refinements. *Health Care Financing Review, 30*(4), 47–59.

Noe, K., & Forgione, D. A. (2014). Economic incentives in the hospice care setting: A comparison of for-profit and nonprofit providers. *Journal of Public Budgeting, Accounting & Financial Management, 26*(2), 233–270. https://doi.org/10.1108/JPBAFM-26-02-2014-B001.

Obermeyer, Z., Makar, M., Abujaber, S., Dominici, F., Block, S., & Cutler, D. M. (2014). Association between the Medicare hospice benefit and health care utilization and costs for patients with poor-prognosis cancer. *Journal of the American Medical Association, 312*(18), 1888–1896. https://doi.org/10.1001/jama.2014.14950.

O'Neill, S. M., Ettner, S. L., & Lorenz, K. A. (2008). Paying the price at the end of life: A consideration of factors that affect the profitability of hospice. *Journal of Palliative Medicine, 11*(7), 1002–1008. https://doi.org/10.1089/jpm.2007.0252.

Orszag, P. R., & Emanuel, E. J. (2010). Health care reform and cost control. *New England Journal of Medicine, 363*(7), 601–603. https://doi.org/10.1056/NEJMp1006571.

Pak, E., Perfetto, C., Yu, Q., & McNabney, M. (2012). Effect of enrollment in the Program of All-Inclusive Care for the Elderly on end-of-life care. *Journal of the American Geriatrics Society, 60*(1), 166–167. https://doi.org/10.1111/j.1532-5415.2011.03745.x.

Rahman, A. N., & Applebaum, R. A. (2009). The nursing home minimum data set assessment instrument: Manifest functions and unintended consequences–past, present, and future. *The Gerontologist, 49*(6), 727–735. https://doi.org/10.1093/geront/gnp066.

Reich, A. D., Hansen, H. B., & Link, B. G. (2016). Fundamental interventions: How clinicians can address the fundamental causes of disease. *Journal of Bioethical Inquiry, 13*(2), 185–192. https://doi.org/10.1007/s11673-016-9715-3.

Rudowitz, R., Garfield, R., & Hinton, E. (2019). *10 things to know about Medicaid: Setting the facts straight.* Henry J. Kaiser Family Foundation. www.kff.org/medicaid/issue-brief/10-things-to-know-about-medicaid-setting-the-facts-straight/.

Sachs, R., & Huberfeld, N. (2019, July 24). The problematic law and policy of Medicaid block grants. *Health Affairs.* www.healthaffairs.org/do/10.1377/hblog20190722.62519/full/.

Saliba, D., Jones, M., Streim, J., Ouslander, J., Berlowitz, D., & Buchanan, J. (2012). Overview of significant changes in the Minimum Data Set for nursing homes version 3.0. *Journal of the American Medical Directors Association, 13*(7), 595–601. https://doi.org/10.1016/j.jamda.2012.06.001.

Schamp, R., & Tenkku, L. (2006). Managed death in a PACE: Pathways in present and advance directives. *Journal of the American Medical Directors Association,* 7(6), 339–344. https://doi.org/10.1016/j.jamda.2006.01.022.

Schoen, C., Osborn, R., Squires, D., Doty, M. M., Pierson, R., & Applebaum, S. (2010). How health insurance design affects access to care and costs, by income, in eleven countries. *Health Affairs, 29*(12), 2323–2334. https://doi.org/10.1377/hlthaff.2010.0862.

Segelman, M., Szydlowski, J., Kinosian, B., McNabney, M., Raziano, D. B., Eng, C., van Reenen, C., & Temkin-Greener, H. (2014). Hospitalizations in the Program of All-Inclusive Care for the Elderly. *Journal of the American Geriatrics Society, 62*(2), 320–324. https://doi.org/10.1111/jgs.12637.

Sinsky, C. A., & Dugdale, D. C. (2013). Medicare payment for cognitive vs procedural care: Minding the gap. *Journal of the American Medical Association Internal Medicine, 173*(18), 1733–1737. https://doi.org/10.1001/jamainternmed.2013.9257.

Sohn, H. (2017). Racial and ethnic disparities in health insurance coverage: Dynamics of gaining and losing coverage over the life-course. *Population Research and Policy Review, 36*(2), 181–201. https://doi.org/10.1007/s11113-016-9416-y.

Sommers, A., & Cohen, M. (2006). *Medicaid's high cost enrollees: How much do they drive program spending?* Henry J. Kaiser Family Foundation. https://kaiserfamilyfoundation.files.wordpress.com/2013/01/7490.pdf.

Stanton, M. W., & Rutherford, M. K. (2005). *The high concentration of U.S. health care expenditures* (No. 06–0060). Agency for Healthcare Research and Quality. https://archive.ahrq.gov/research/findings/factsheets/costs/expriach/.

Stokes, J., Panagioti, M., Alam, R., Checkland, K., Cheraghi-Sohi, S., & Bower, P. (2015). Effectiveness of case management for "at risk" patients in primary care: A systematic review and meta-analysis. *PLoS ONE*. http://journals.plos.org/plosone/article?id=10.1371/journal.pone.0132340.

Temkin-Greener, H., & Mukamel, D. B. (2002). Predicting place of death in the program of all-inclusive care for the elderly (PACE): Participant versus program characteristics. *Journal of the American Geriatrics Society, 50*(1), 125–135.

Teno, J. M., Gozalo, P. L., Bynum, J. P. W., Leland, N. E., Miller, S. C., Morden, N. E., Scupp, T., Goodman, D. C., & Mor, V. (2013). Change in end-of-life care for Medicare beneficiaries: Site of death, place of care, and health care transitions in 2000, 2005, and 2009. *Journal of the American Medical Association, 309*(5), 470. https://doi.org/10.1001/jama.2012.207624.

Thompson, J. W., Carlson, M. D. A., & Bradley, E. H. (2012). U.S. hospice industry experienced considerable turbulence from changes in ownership, growth, and shift to for-profit status. *Health Affairs, 31*(6), 1286–1293. https://doi.org/10.1377/hlthaff.2011.1247.

Thompson, S., & Oliver, D. P. (2008). A new model for long-term care: Balancing palliative and restorative care delivery. *Journal of Housing For the Elderly, 22*(3), 169–194. https://doi.org/10.1080/02763890802232014.

U.S. Census Bureau. (2017). *Health insurance coverage in the United States: 2016*. www.census.gov/library/publications/2017/demo/p60-260.html.

Unroe, K. T., Sachs, G. A., Dennis, M. E., Hickman, S. E., Stump, T. E., Tu, W., & Callahan, C. M. (2016). Effect of hospice use on costs of care for long-stay nursing home decedents. *Journal of the American Geriatrics Society, 64*(4), 723–730. https://doi.org/10.1111/jgs.14070.

Wachterman, M. W., Hailpern, S. M., Keating, N. L., Tamura, M. K., & O'Hare, A. M. (2018). Association between hospice length of stay, health care utilization, and Medicare costs at the end of life among patients who received maintenance hemodialysis. *Journal of the American Medical Association Internal Medicine, 178*(6), 792–799. https://doi.org/10.1001/jamainternmed.2018.0256.

Wachterman, M.W., Marcantonio, E. R., Davis, R. B., & McCarthy, E. P. (2011). Association of hospice agency profit status with patient diagnosis, location of care, and length of stay. *Journal of the American Medical Association, 305*(5), 472–479. https://doi.org/10.1001/jama.2011.70.

Wallace, J., & Song, Z. (2016). Traditional Medicare versus private insurance: How spending, volume, and price change at age sixty-five. *Health Affairs, 35*(5), 864–872. https://doi.org/10.1377/hlthaff.2015.1195.

Wang, S., Hsu, S. H., Huang, S., Soulos, P. R., & Gross, C. P. (2017). Longer periods of hospice service associated with lower end-of-life spending in regions with high expenditures. *Health Affairs, 36*(2), 328–336. https://doi.org/10.1377/hlthaff.2016.0683.

Watts, M. O., Musumeci, M., & Chidambaram, P. (2020). *Medicaid home and community-based services enrollment and spending* (No. 9294–02). Kaiser Family Foundation. www.kff.org/report-section/medicaid-home-and-community-based-services-enrollment-and-spending-issue-brief/.

Weinstein, M. C., & Skinner, J. A. (2010). Comparative effectiveness and health care spending – Implications for reform. *New England Journal of Medicine, 362*(5), 460–465. https://doi.org/10.1056/NEJMsb0911104.

Wiener, J. M., & Tilly, J. (2003). End-of-life care in the United States: Policy issues and model programs of integrated care. *International Journal of Integrated Care, 3*. www.ncbi.nlm.nih.gov/pmc/articles/PMC1483949/.

Wysocki, A., Butler, M., Kane, R. L., Kane, R. A., Shippee, T., & Sainfort, F. (2012). *Long-term care for older adults: A review of home and community-based services versus institutional care* (12(13)-EHC134-EF; Comparative Effectiveness Reviews, No. 81). Agency for Healthcare Research and Quality (US). www.ncbi.nlm.nih.gov/books/NBK114863/.

Zuckerman, R. B., Stearns, S. C., & Sheingold, S. H. (2016). Hospice use, hospitalization, and Medicare spending at the end of life. *The Journals of Gerontology: Series B, 71*(3), 569–580. https://doi.org/10.1093/geronb/gbv109.

Zuckerman, S., Williams, A. F., & Stockley, K. E. (2009). Trends in Medicaid physician fees, 2003–2008. *Health Affairs, 28*(3), w510–w519. https://doi.org/10.1377/hlthaff.28.3.w510.

7
ADVANCE CARE PLANNING

People can plan ahead for a predictable death. That is, patients and their families have a lot of information about what their final weeks and days will be like, and they can make medical decisions in anticipation. Thus the judicial system of the United States now has decades of precedent for handling both routine and unusual circumstances that arise around predictable deaths. Routine circumstances include multiple decisions about care, often for a patient who no longer has the legal competence to make choices. In unusual circumstances, family members and/or health care professionals may go to court to contest the right to make a medical decision.

In this chapter, I first sketch out the model of patient autonomy that is the basis for law. I go on to describe the process of advance care planning, which is a method for making medical decisions before they need to be implemented. Patients can use advance care planning to request treatments, and also to elect to forgo or stop treatments. I describe sociohistorical disparities in access to and use of these legal precedents. Finally, I analyze how well current laws represent and anticipate the medical situations that people face in practice, and how well they model the decision-making process as it truly occurs.

Patient Autonomy in End-of-Life Planning

Before death was predictable, health care was doctor-directed: The doctor had the specialized knowledge and expertise necessary to make decisions about the patient's care, and it was incumbent upon the doctor to use his or her powers for the patient's good (Will, 2011a). This system was paternalistic, such that patients had no choice but to trust the doctor to preserve their best interests. Doctors even practiced benevolent deception, lying or omitting information when interacting with the patient if they thought it best (Will, 2011a).

Around 1900, the epidemiological transition made deaths more predictable. Other changes occurred in the health care system as well. Patients began to receive care in clinics or hospitals rather than in their own home, they began to receive care from multiple doctors and an expanding number of other types of health care professionals, and clinicians began to rely on diagnostic tests, rather than examination of the patient, to determine the patient's medical problem (Will, 2011b). Health insurance emerged as a new industry, one that added a third party to the doctor–patient relationship (Maioni, 1998). These changes made the doctor–patient relationship increasingly impersonal. This distance between doctor and patient likely made it more difficult for doctors to understand the patient's social context and hence, his or her best interests.

At the same time, U.S. courts were defining informed consent (Randall & Downie, 2006). In this line of thought, the inherent dignity of persons gives them the right to make their own moral decisions. Consent in medicine means that the doctor and patient jointly investigate alternative courses of action, rather than that the patient simply acquiesces to the doctor's wishes (Randall & Downie, 2006). The role of the doctor is to advise the patient, providing him or her with sufficient accurate information to allow the patient to determine what happens to him or her. The revelations of physician abuses of power during World War II further reinforced the value of informed consent, as did the Civil Rights Era focus on self-determination (Hunter, 2010).

Thus, modern end-of-life law in the U.S. is intended to check the power of doctors and preserve patient self-determination, even after the patient has lost decision-making capacity. At least three out of ten older people lack the capacity to make an important medical decision for themselves in the last days of life (Raymont et al., 2004; Silveira et al., 2010). In this era of informed consent, legally competent patients can appoint a surrogate to preserve their self-determination after they lose competence. The legal standard for surrogate decision-making is *substituted judgment* (Pope, 2012). By this standard, surrogates make the decision that they believe the patient would have made, if able. Surrogates are not, in ordinary circumstances, legally permitted to follow their own judgment for what is in the best interests of the patient. The goal is to preserve the patient's legal autonomy, rather than for the surrogate to serve as a guardian or overseer.

This priority on autonomy sets the life course principle of agency at odds with the life course principle of linked lives (Elder et al., 2003). That is, the law preserves an individual's agency as though individuals are independent and isolated legal entities, when in fact people depend upon, and are responsible for, various other people. Bioethicists have noted that ideally, the law should honor not only autonomy, but also values such as welfare (Bruce et al., 2016). Nevertheless, the law does prioritize autonomy, in such a way that poses a variety of challenges to doctors, patients, and families.

Legal Documents

Under law, competent adults may exercise their autonomy by completing advance directives, which are signed and witnessed documents that address medical care in a future period of incompetence. States, rather than the federal government, have jurisdiction over this area of law, and so consistent nationwide rules neither exist now nor are likely to emerge in the future (Olick, 2012). Thus, I describe advance care planning broadly, as it applies in many or most states. Readers interested in completing their own advance care plans, or in better understanding local conditions, should consult the laws of their state.[1]

Advance directives include the living will and the durable power of attorney for health care. A living will describes the treatments a person would and would not want if dying and incapacitated. Individuals have the right to refuse medical treatment; but at the same time, health care professionals act under the law of constructive or implied consent. Constructive consent is the assumption that incapacitated patients would choose to live rather than to die, and accordingly would choose to receive all possible medical treatment. Human rights lawyer Luis Kutner (1968) first questioned this assumption in the legal literature, noting that there should be some mechanism for individuals to be able to exercise their right to refuse treatment even when incapacitated. He proposed the living will.

Therefore, people who want all possible treatments do not, technically, need to complete a living will, and most people use the living will as a means of refusing interventions (Winter & Parks, 2012b). However, people who want all possible treatments may complete a living will to establish their preferences clearly for their family members and health care professionals. The living will can also make clear situations in which people would like to receive some treatments but refuse others.

The living will has three key shortcomings. First, for a living will to be effective, people need to be able to accurately predict the medical circumstances of their deaths. The treatments that apply to one condition may not apply to another (Alonso et al., 2017). For example, a cancer patient may complete a living will with thorough instructions regarding cancer care, but if she is subsequently the victim of a car accident, cancer care is not the type of care she will require. Even when patients correctly predict their circumstances, the human brain is very poor at predicting what the future will feel like. Just as it is difficult to pack the right clothes for a tropical vacation in the middle of a New England winter, it is difficult for relatively healthy people to know what care will be most important to them in their last days of life (Loewenstein, 2005; Winter et al., 2009).

Second, for a living will to be effective, a person needs to have sufficient health literacy to write specific, applicable provisions. Most people have broad values and goals, such as not being a burden to others, but they do not know what specific steps a health care provider might take to achieve those goals (Winter, 2013). Unfortunately, health care providers do not know, either, since concepts such as burden are qualitative (Nauck et al., 2014). Lawyers frequently write living wills on behalf of their clients, because the living will needs to be properly executed to be legally binding. Lawyers do not solve the health literacy problem, however, since most lawyers are not especially familiar with medical practice. The reader might also note that problems one and two are mutually reinforcing, insofar as a living will ought neither be too general nor too specific.

Third, for a living will to be effective, health care professionals need to have it at the time of treatment. Many people complete a living will and then lovingly preserve it with other their valuable records, such as in a bank safe deposit box, where no one can get to it quickly in an emergency. Some health systems have invested in electronic medical records that are available to any provider or hospital within the system. However, electronic medical records are proprietary software packages that are usually incompatible with one another, such that living wills are not available if a person experiences a medical crisis outside of his or her health care system. There is no nationwide system of medical records, as other nations such as France use to good effect.

Researchers and policymakers have been publishing these critiques of the living will in prominent journals for decades (Eisendrath & Jonsen, 1983; Fagerlin & Schneider, 2004; Shapiro, 2015; Tonelli, 1996). Yet living wills remain well established in U.S. law. Advance directives can take another form, the durable power of attorney for health care (DPAHC), which may compensate for some of the weaknesses of living wills. This law transfers legal decision-making ability from an incapacitated patient to a surrogate or proxy decision-maker. Many states automatically designate one's next-of-kin, usually a spouse or adult child, to serve as the DPAHC. This designation is consistent with the preferences of the vast majority of individuals (Carr & Khodyakov, 2007b). In states without a default assignment, or to override a state's default assignment, individuals can complete legal forms nominating a DPAHC. Overwhelmingly, people choose a family member because they believe that family members are the appropriate parties to make such a decision in a moral and ethical sense, and because they believe that their family knows their wishes best (Kelly et al., 2012).

However, like the living will, the DPAHC comes with several obvious problems. First, the laws assume that the dying person has a nuclear family unit. Health care providers and the law both struggle with care delivery for incapacitated patients who lack immediate family such as a spouse and adult children (Cohen et al., 2015). Such patients tend to experience life-prolonging treatment during long hospital stays, and the people who make decisions for these patients rarely have any notion of what the patient would have wanted (Weiss et al., 2012). Still other people have family, but family is becoming increasingly complex. For example, the divorce rate among adults over the age of 50 has doubled since 1990 (Brown et al., 2019). Adult children from multiple unions, plus partners from multiple unions, may comprise a dying person's family, making decision-making authority uncertain. The DPAHC is a good option both for people who lack family and for people who have large and complex families, but patients in these situations are less likely than others to appoint one, perhaps because they too are at a loss for whom to choose (Moorman & Boerner, 2018).

Moreover, decision-making often stirs up family discord (Boelk & Kramer, 2012). In some cases, the discord is ongoing and long-standing, and a dying family member simply further exacerbates the situation. Some people are estranged from family members, or have experienced neglect or abuse in those relationships (Kong & Moorman, 2015). In other cases, family members have a peaceable past, but disagree specifically about the end-of-life decision to be made and who should make it, and they have poor communication. Such cases sometimes reach courts of law (Quill, 2005), and although the courts adjudicate who has the right to make decisions for the patient, it seems unlikely that a legal solution would reduce conflict in the family.

A second major problem with the DPAHC, although it has received less attention in research, is the potential burden it may place on surrogates. In theory, there should be little to no burden because the surrogate is not truly making a decision, but rather simply relating or reporting a decision the patient has already made (Braun et al., 2009). In practice, surrogates do not experience their role in this way; rather, they feel responsible for the life or death of the patient (Schenker et al., 2012). Serving as a surrogate is very emotionally distressing, with some surrogates feeling guilt and doubt for years after the death, and some experiencing clinical problems such as post-traumatic stress or complicated grief (Wendler & Rid, 2011). Surrogates cope better when they feel certain that they are doing what the patient wanted (Braun et al., 2008). Surrogates who know they followed the patient's preferences fare better in the aftermath of the death than do surrogates who did not know what the patient wanted (Vig et al., 2007).

The third apparent problem with the DPAHC concerns the standard of substituted judgment. Patients feel quite sure that their family members understand their wishes, especially when they have strong relationships with those family members (Moorman, 2011b). However, two lines of research suggest that family members do not always understand wishes. One line of research poses hypothetical end-of-life scenarios to would-be patients and their chosen surrogates, asks both to choose a treatment for the patient, and then compares answers. For example, a hypothetical scenario may be that the patient is in pain, or that the patient has advanced dementia. Surrogate decisions often do not match the patient's choice even when the decision is a broad one between stopping or continuing life-prolonging treatment (Moorman & Carr, 2008; Moorman & Inoue, 2013; Parks et al., 2011; Shalowitz et al., 2006).

A second line of research interviews surrogates who have made decisions. Surrogates do not have a uniform understanding of their role (Lilley et al., 2017), and they list many factors that affected their decisions in addition to the patient's preferences (Fritch et al., 2013; Vig et al., 2006). Most surrogates say that the patient's well-being, rather than the patient's preferences, was the major factor driving their decision (Devnani et al., 2017). Together, studies using these two very different methods converge in indicating that surrogates often cannot or do not achieve substituted judgment.

There is a group of older persons who value independence and self-determination, and so want a strict substituted judgment (Moorman, 2011a). However, the standard of substituted judgment oversimplifies what many patients desire from a DPAHC. For example, there are patients who wish to make their own decisions, and want them followed strictly, but not to preserve their autonomy so much as to spare others the burden (McPherson et al., 2007a; Winter & Parks, 2012a). Many dying people spend a great deal of time worrying about being, or becoming, a burden to others, and it is a significant source of suffering for them (McPherson et al., 2007b). Some patients respond by giving the surrogate complete latitude to make the decision (Terry et al., 1999), while others respond by eliminating the decision for the surrogate by making it themselves. Surrogates do fare better in their bereavement when their task was to report a patient's clear preference rather than to discern what the patient would have wanted (Braun et al., 2008, 2009). However, patients frequently overestimate the extent to which their care is burdensome to others, and so the psychosocial well-being of this group of burden-sensitive patients might be higher if they were in fact *less* independent in their decision-making (McPherson et al., 2007b).

At the other extreme, some patients simply do not place high value on self-determination, either in medical decision-making in general, or in the end-of-life context in particular. Some patients find medical decision-making to be burdensome to the extent that they would prefer that someone else do it (Wolff & Boyd, 2015). Other people are content for a surrogate's preferences to override their own in an end-of-life situation, reasoning that the survivors will have to live with the sense of moral responsibility for how the death occurred (Terry et al., 1999).

Still other people view the family, rather than the self, as the decision-making unit (Chan, 2004; Ho, 2008). They value family-determination instead of self-determination. That is, a decision that did not account for family opinions and the well-being of the family would not be a truly autonomous one. Ho (2008, p. 128) calls this "relational autonomy" and traces it from lines of feminist thought, while Chan (2004, p. 95) calls this the "connected self" and traces it to Confucian thought. Both argue that requiring a patient to select treatments without his or her family's input, when in fact that patient desires family input, is a violation of the patient's rights.

Yet another group of patients see their appointment of a DPAHC, rather than their selection of treatments, as their primary exercise in autonomy. Here, the focus is not adherence to a treatment choice that the patient made in advance, but rather adherence to the way in which the patient wanted the decision to be made (Brudney, 2009). They trust the surrogate to make a decision as he or she sees fit when the times comes, and would be upset if their surrogate did not make the decision – for example, if a physician made a treatment choice unilaterally without consulting the surrogate (Teno et al., 2011).

Finally, a group of patients thinks that the way the decision should be made depends on the circumstances. Fins and colleagues (2005) distinguish between a contractual approach to advance directives, where surrogates carry out the patient's preferences strictly, and a covenantal approach, where the patient has granted the surrogate agency to come to decisions. In that study, both patients and their intended surrogates viewed a preference for no treatment as a contract that the surrogate is required to uphold, an area for strict substituted judgment. But they saw a preference for all treatment as a covenant, contingent on the surrogate's observations of the patient's well-being and likely outcomes (Fins et al., 2005). That is, the patient trusts the surrogate to be able to identify the point at which further treatment is futile and burdensome, and to be able to defend the patient's best interests at that time.

Discussions

Scholars and clinicians counter these many problems with the living will and DPAHC by asserting that advance directive completion was never meant to occur in a vacuum, but rather along with discussions with surrogates, other family members, and health care providers. The living will and DPAHC are legally binding records, but discussion is equally, if not more, important. Discussions are opportunities for health care providers to convey information about specific treatments, and they are opportunities for surrogate decision-makers to better understand patient preferences. Moreover, discussions should be repeated, and formal plans should be revisited, as the patient's circumstances change and as state-of-the-art treatment changes, because although patients' overall values remain stable, their preferences regarding specific treatments develop over time (Ditto et al., 2006; Pruchno et al., 2008). A challenge here is that Medicare reimburses physicians for just 60 minutes of conversation about advanced care planning with each patient, and any further discussions go unpaid (Doukas, 2017). Even this single reimbursement was the result of a highly politicized process in the early 2010s, where conservative politicians were concerned that advance care planning constituted rationing of care for older persons (Tinetti, 2012).

Further, the evidence on discussions is equivocal. Some research indicates that discussions do nothing: Multiple studies document that family discussions about advance care planning do not improve surrogates' substituted judgment in hypothetical scenario tasks (Shalowitz et al., 2006). Many patient–surrogate pairs even disagree about whether they have ever discussed the patient's preferences (Fried et al., 2017). Physicians report that their discussions with a patient do not change their fundamental orientation towards decision-making for that patient (Torke et al., 2010).

Other research indicates that discussions improve the chances that a dying person will receive goal-concordant care (Mack et al., 2010). Discussion works best when it is structured and mediated by a trained nurse, social worker, or other clinician (L. L. Emanuel et al., 1995). Clinicians have developed a number of decision aids to help patients and families think through decision-making together and communicate with health care providers (Butler et al., 2014), and some health care systems have successfully implemented facilitated advance care planning programs for their sickest patients (Kirchhoff et al., 2012).

The debate about the success of discussions is part of a broader debate about whether advance care planning achieves its goals, given the many well-documented problems with living wills, DPAHCs, and discussions. Systematic reviews indicate that advance care planning does reduce hospitalizations and increase the use of hospice, resulting in lower levels of life-prolonging treatment (Brinkman-Stoppelenburg et al., 2014; Khandelwal et al., 2015; Teno et al., 2007). Few studies in the U.S. to date employ an experimental design, which poses a problem for assessment: Likely, the people who complete advance care planning are not random, but rather are people who have material resources and are pro-active regarding their health. However, the randomized controlled trials that do exist have shown benefits, for example, to substituted judgment and to the grief process of surrogates (Song et al., 2015). Editorials calling for its demise are likely to continue, but incremental efforts to improve advance care planning seem more likely to bear fruit.

This evidence suggests that ongoing efforts to encourage people to complete advance care plans are not wasted. In 1990, the U.S. Congress institutionalized the practice of advance care planning nationally by passing the Patient Self-Determination Act (PSDA). Under this law, all medical facilities that receive federal funding are required to inform patients of their right to complete advance care planning. The law did immediately boost rates of planning, although overall rates of planning remained low (E. J. Emanuel et al., 1993; Teno et al., 1997). The best estimate in about 2015 was that about one-third of U.S. adults had formal advance care plans (Yadav et al., 2017). The proportion of older adults who had them was much higher, at three-quarters (Harrison et al., 2016; Silveira et al., 2014). Discussions lagged somewhat behind, with 60% of older adults reporting that they had discussed their preferences with someone (Kale et al., 2016). Simply put, people need to know how and why advance care planning is important in their own lives before they will complete it (Schickedanz et al., 2009). Therefore, life events such as the death of a loved one or one's own hospitalization spur people to plan (Carr, 2012c; Carr & Khodyakov, 2007a; Fried et al., 2009). Facing one's own death is unpleasant and uncomfortable, and people will not – perhaps cannot, psychologically – do it without sufficient impetus (Fried et al., 2010).

Physician Orders for Life-Sustaining Treatment

Because most people in the U.S. today have a predictable death, advance directives do not need to do all the work of advance care planning. That is, advance directives can be anticipatory steps that prepare patients and surrogates to be ready to make medical decisions when the time arrives (Sudore, 2010). They are a mechanism to begin the process of articulating a patient's values and developing his or her treatment preferences (Fried et al., 2009, 2010). Then, new mechanisms can do the work of informing health care providers about specific treatments for a known condition in advance of crisis. For example, physician orders for life-sustaining treatment (POLST) is gaining nationwide acceptance. POLST originated in Oregon in 1991, was available in 12 states by 2010, and was under development in some form in all states and Washington, D.C., by 2018 (Karp & Sabatino, 2011).[2] POLST is an additional step of advance care planning that follows completion of advance directives. A POLST establishes a set of standing medical orders for seriously ill people (National POLST Paradigm, 2019). Specifically, POLST creates a patient-specific plan for cardiopulmonary resuscitation (CPR), hospital and intensive care unit (ICU) admission, mechanical ventilation, and artificial nutrition or hydration.

A rule of thumb is that if the health care provider would not be surprised were the patient to die within the next year, then the time is right to complete POLST. At that point, health care providers, patients, and surrogates can talk in concrete terms about possible end-of-life scenarios. The health care provider, rather than the patient, completes the POLST, includes it in the patient's medical record, and is accountable for following it. A key aspect of POLST is that emergency medical technicians (EMTs) can use it in an emergency, whereas they cannot use advance directives.

Much of the empirical research on POLST comes from Oregon, which has had POLST the longest. Large-scale studies show benefits. For example, POLST increases the probability of dying where one wants (Fromme et al., 2014) and of receiving treatment consistent with one's preferences (Hickman et al., 2010). Yet, some argue that there is not yet a sufficient base of evidence to warrant the rapid expansion of POLST, that the mechanisms for amending one's POLST are not adequately developed, and that physicians do not always understand POLST forms correctly (Moore et al., 2016). There is also an ongoing debate in medical journals concerning potential amendments to the POLST form, language, and use, such as whether a single, national form is possible and whether all people over the age of 80 should complete one (Hickman et al., 2017; Stuart & Thielke, 2017, 2018). Likely, POLST will undergo revisions and refinements in the future, but it is now a well-established part of end-of-life care that is likely to become even more widely used.

Social Disparities in Advance Care Planning

There are sharp social differences in who does and does not complete advance care plans. Sexual orientation is one such social dividing line, although very little empirical research on this topic appeared before approximately 2013 (Buckey & Browning, 2013).

There is a long history of discrimination against lesbian, gay, bisexual, and transgender (LGBT) persons in healthcare, which is compounded by the fact that LGBT persons tend to have greater health care needs than their heterosexual peers because of the effects of the discrimination they experience in daily life (Office of Disease Prevention and Health Promotion, 2019). Therefore, unpartnered LGBT persons, especially transgender men and women, may be less likely than heterosexual persons to have completed advance care plans because they have less contact with health care services, and because they may be without the nuclear family that advance care planning assumes (Brennan-Ing et al., 2014; Kcomt & Gorey, 2017).

However, partnered LGBT individuals are *more* likely than heterosexual persons to have completed advance care plans, perhaps because they have a partner to advocate for them in the health care system and with their families (Buckey & Browning, 2013). Heterosexual individuals can afford to pay relatively little attention to advance care plans, because the laws of most states protect immediate family as decision-makers. LGBT individuals devote more time to their living wills, DPAHCs, and discussions *because* the laws of most states protect immediate family as decision-makers (Buckey & Browning, 2013). That is, LGBT individuals may be concerned that members of their families of origin would make medical decisions that they would not make for themselves as patients, or that their families would contest the right of partners and other non-relatives to make decisions on their behalf. Spouses have first right to make decisions in many states, and same-sex marriage is legal in the U.S. However, this right is newly won and same-sex couples feel uncertain about the future stability of legal protections (Thomeer et al., 2017). Further, observers note that the *existence* of legal protections is distinct from the *enforcement* of legal protections, such that discrimination is likely to continue to occur despite its unlawfulness (Marsack & Stephenson, 2017; Wahlert & Fiester, 2013).

Most health care professionals lack knowledge about how to address end-of-life with LGBT patients, although they do it with greater success after they receive training in LGBT health issues (Carabez & Scott, 2016; Porter & Krinsky, 2014). Professional organizations of service providers, especially social workers, are developing standards for the competencies providers should have to practice effectively with LGBT older adults (Fredriksen-Goldsen et al., 2014). The National Center on LGBT Aging provides a number of resources to aging service providers, including free training materials (SAGE Advocacy and Services for LGBT Elders, 2019).

A second social factor that shapes disparities in advance care planning is race and ethnicity. People of color in the U.S. complete plans at much lower rates than do White Americans (Garrido et al., 2014; Harrison et al., 2016). Some of these differences are due to racism in access to and quality of care, as well as the poorer socioeconomic position of many persons of color (Carr, 2012b; Johnson et al., 2008). There are also group differences in familiarity with advance care planning, with Hispanics particularly unlikely to be aware of advance care planning as an option (Carr, 2012a).

However, advance care plans are also inconsistent with some religious or spiritual beliefs about the nature of death, and with some cultural practices surrounding decision-making. For example, informal discussions may be especially effective planning among Hispanic Americans (Shen et al., 2016). Many Hispanics see advance care planning as a family issue and find the DPAHC, which appoints a single surrogate, to be off-putting (Kelley et al., 2010; Kwak & Haley, 2005). Blacks are more likely than Whites to turn to their religious or spiritual beliefs to help them cope with death (True et al., 2005). Black Protestant congregations tend to believe that God has a plan for one's death, with which humans ought not interfere (Carr, 2011; Garrido et al., 2013). Several South Asian religions teach passive acceptance in the face of death, such that church-based interventions may be likely to promote advance care planning most effectively (Biondo et al., 2017; Sun et al., 2017).

Disparities are not set in stone, but rather change alongside alterations in the health care system, health education, health policy, and so forth (Portanova et al., 2017). There is some evidence that increasing numbers of Blacks are completing advance care plans, for instance (Koss & Baker, 2017). Moreover, people have intersecting characteristics that affect the disparities they face, for example, being both Black and LGBT (Kim et al., 2017). Therefore, the message to take away from this section is that the facilitators of and barriers to advance care planning are related not only to personal choices, but also to systemic social patterns of advantage and disadvantage.

Control, Decision-Making, and Systemic Change

The evolution of advance care planning thus far suggests two areas for improvement that draw upon multiple disciplines. First, bioethicists and social scientists focus on the narrative frames in which autonomy and death currently sit, as well as ways to reframe these ideas in the future to make the decision-making process easier for patients, families, and health care providers alike. Second, legal scholars and philosophers focus on how the law might better support stakeholders in end-of-life decision-making by better reflecting the real situations that people face rather than unattainable ideals. These approaches contribute useful ideas for the next generation of advance care planning.

First, some medical ethicists argue that patient autonomy has come to have an increasingly transactional meaning whereby patients have the right to whatever medical services they request (Randall & Downie, 2006). The transactional conception of autonomy developed from free market economics, where the patient is a consumer of health care services. Transactional autonomy grants the patient a certain moral independence from the doctor, on the assumption that the doctor should have no say in determining what is good for the patient. If the patient, or the patient's insurance, can pay, then the doctor's responsibility is to provide, even if the choice runs counter to the doctor's professional opinion or moral judgment. For example, under transactional autonomy, a patient who requests a non-beneficial treatment should receive it, even if the doctor views the treatment as a waste of resources that will harm the patient.

Ethicists object to the transactional form of autonomy on several grounds (Randall & Downie, 2006). First, completely excluding the doctor from decision-making impinges on the doctor's own autonomy and expertise. Because doctor bears both legal and moral responsibility for the patient's outcomes, the doctor should have some input into treatment decisions. Some physicians have even suggested that transactional autonomy allows doctors to renege their duty to dying patients, essentially abandoning patients to make medical decisions without guidance or support (Loewy, 2005). Second, the health care market is unlike the free market in that money in health care is often a common good derived from taxpayer funding or an insurance pool rather than the patient's own property. Therefore, use of those resources requires input from people beyond the patient him or herself. Third, in decision-making, patients assume responsibilities as well as rights. Autonomy should mean that an individual is free to choose while considering effects on others, not only immediate effects on the self. Therefore, advance care planning is misdirected if it is viewed as a list of patient demands that the doctor is obligated to follow to the letter. Several of the criticisms of advance directives – for example, the debate about specific, applicable provisions vs. broad values and goals – assume that autonomy is essentially transactional. A more appropriate division of labor between doctor and patient may be to consider the patient to be the expert on his or her own values and preferences, and to consider the doctor to be the expert on how to use medicine to realize those values and preferences (Billings & Krakauer, 2011).

Moreover, bioethicists argue that autonomy is illusory (Drought & Koenig, 2002). Although people like to believe that death is under the control of medicine and can be postponed indefinitely, this is false (Conrad, 2014). Therefore, the choices there are to make and the autonomy to be exercised are extremely circumscribed when someone is dying. My friend once said of her toddler's autonomy: He can climb into the car seat himself, or Mommy can put him in the car seat, but either way, he has to get into the car seat. This example illustrates two important points about the end of life. First, death, like the car seat, is inevitable. So why emphasize autonomy and decision-making as though they were rational processes that meaningfully affect the ultimate outcome (Lynn et al., 2000)? There is no reason for surrogates to carry years of guilt for choosing, for example, to stop life-prolonging treatment, because the surrogate is not responsible for choosing the patient's death (Braun et al., 2009). Many of the decisions surrogates agonize over concern a difference of only hours of life. One straightforward way of producing culture change in advance care planning may be to change the clinical language surrounding the end of treatment. For example, terms like *allow natural death* are much more palatable than terms like *do not resuscitate* (Fairlie, 2017).

To return briefly to the car seat example, there is another point to be made about the nature of autonomy at the end of life, which is that process matters. The child cares enormously about whether he gets into the car seat himself or whether Mommy helps him. That decision affects his sense of control and his overall feelings about himself, even if the result – riding in the car seat – is the same either way. The end of life is analogous. Patients, survivors, and medical professionals all care about whether the death feels good or bad (Steinhauser et al., 2000). The details of whether the patient feels like a burden to others and whether the surrogate believes the physician listened to her concerns, for example, matter a great deal. Control over these details is the autonomy that patients want.

In line with this last concern is research considering how the law might better serve the real processes by which decisions are made at the end of life. Several medical ethicists argue that substituted judgment should be abandoned as the standard for surrogates because, given how rarely a true substituted judgment is possible in practice, continuing to rely on a flawed standard is not ethical (Torke et al., 2008). Autonomy is only one of several important values that patients and families hold (Ikonomidis & Singer, 1999). In fact, some believe that there are other concerns more important than autonomy (Bruce et al., 2016). Perhaps a better decision-making standard than substituted judgment is "best judgment," or honoring the surrogate's love for the patient, which includes both the patient's autonomy as a unique person and also his or her welfare as a member of humankind (Stonestreet, 2014, p. 523). Surrogates would be responsible neither for knowing what the patient would have wanted nor for giving their own opinion about treatment. Instead, the surrogate would be the expert on the patient's values and preferences, while the doctor would be the expert on the types of medical care that would be congruent with that person's vision of a good death (Sulmasy & Snyder, 2010). This model is consistent with ethical models of decisional sharing between competent patients and their physicians (Billings & Krakauer, 2011). The surrogate's job is simply to speak for the patient.

Summary

In the U.S., people have the right to accept or refuse medical treatment. This right becomes complicated for dying people, perhaps 30% of whom lack the capacity to make medical decisions. Advance care planning is the legal mechanism in place to allow incapacitated individuals to accept or refuse treatment. Advance care planning has three parts: a living will, a durable power of attorney for health care, and informal discussions with family and health care providers. Each of these three parts has serious limitations; however, people who do all three parts and repeat and amend them over time have better deaths than people who do more limited planning. Concrete POLST plans in the last year of life may reinforce advance care planning.

Important social disparities in advance care planning exist, especially by sexual orientation and by race/ethnicity. Sexual and gender minorities have high rates of planning when they are partnered, but single LGBT people are unlikely to plan. Health care need tends to be high in the LGBT population, and ability to rely on next-of-kin, low, such that they are a vulnerable group of older adults. Americans of color are less likely to be aware of advance care planning than White Americans, and less likely to complete planning even when they are aware. Elements of advance care planning law, such as the ability to appoint only one DPAHC, are inconsistent with the cultural practices that some communities observe at the end of life.

Accepting or refusing medical treatment is a matter of autonomy, or self-determination. A transactional approach to autonomy emphasizes the patient as a customer whose wishes are always most important. A broader approach to autonomy reduces some of the problems with advance care planning, because it acknowledges the patient's responsibilities, as well as the roles of health care providers and family members in decision-making. Interdisciplinary contributions to advance care planning reform seem likely to improve upon the successes of advance care planning for future cohorts.

Notes

1. Forms for each state are available at: www.aarp.org/caregiving/financial-legal/free-printable-advance-directives/.
2. The name of this mechanism differs from state to state, with synonyms including medical orders for life-sustaining treatment (MOLST); physician orders for scope of treatment (POST); and medical orders for scope of treatment (MOST).

References

Alonso, A., Dörr, D., & Szabo, K. (2017). Critical appraisal of advance directives given by patients with fatal acute stroke: An observational cohort study. *BMC Medical Ethics, 18*, 7. https://doi.org/10.1186/s12910-016-0166-5.

Billings, J. A., & Krakauer, E. L. (2011). On patient autonomy and physician responsibility in end-of-life care. *Archives of Internal Medicine, 171*(9), 849–853. https://doi.org/10.1001/archinternmed.2011.180.

Biondo, P. D., Kalia, R., Khan, R., Asghar, N., Banerjee, C., Boulton, D., Marlett, N., Shklarov, S., & Simon, J. E. (2017). Understanding advance care planning within the South Asian community. *Health Expectations, 20*(5), 911–919. https://doi.org/10.1111/hex.12531.

Boelk, A. Z., & Kramer, B. J. (2012). Advancing theory of family conflict at the end of life: A hospice case study. *Journal of Pain and Symptom Management, 44*(5), 655–670. https://doi.org/10.1016/j.jpainsymman.2011.11.004.

Braun, U. K., Beyth, R. J., Ford, M. E., & McCullough, L. B. (2008). Voices of African American, Caucasian, and Hispanic surrogates on the burdens of end-of-life decision making. *Journal of General Internal Medicine, 23*(3), 267–274. https://doi.org/10.1007/s11606-007-0487-7.

Braun, U. K., Naik, A. D., & McCullough, L. B. (2009). Reconceptualizing the experience of surrogate decision making: Reports vs genuine decisions. *The Annals of Family Medicine*, 7(3), 249–253. https://doi.org/10.1370/afm.963.

Brennan-Ing, M., Seidel, L., Larson, B., & Karpiak, S. E. (2014). Social care networks and older LGBT adults: Challenges for the future. *Journal of Homosexuality*, *61*(1), 21–52. https://doi.org/10.1080/00918369.2013.835235.

Brinkman-Stoppelenburg, A., Rietjens, J. A., & van der Heide, A. (2014). The effects of advance care planning on end-of-life care: A systematic review. *Palliative Medicine*, *28*(8), 1000–1025. https://doi.org/10.1177/0269216314526272.

Brown, S. L., Lin, I.-F., Hammersmith, A. M., & Wright, M. R. (2019). Repartnering following gray divorce: The roles of resources and constraints for women and men. *Demography*, *56*(2), 503–523. https://doi.org/10.1007/s13524-018-0752-x.

Bruce, C. R., Bibler, T., Childress, A. M., Stephens, A. L., Pena, A. M., & Allen, N. G. (2016). Navigating ethical conflicts between advance directives and surrogate decision-makers' interpretations of patient wishes. *Chest*, *149*(2), 562–567. https://doi.org/10.1378/chest.15-2209.

Brudney, D. (2009). Beyond autonomy and best interests. *Hastings Center Report*, *39*(2), 31–37. https://doi.org/10.1353/hcr.0.0113.

Buckey, J. W., & Browning, C. N. (2013). Factors affecting the LGBT population when choosing a surrogate decision maker. *Journal of Social Service Research*, *39*(2), 233–252. https://doi.org/10.1080/01488376.2012.754205.

Butler, M., Ratner, E., McCreedy, E., Shippee, N., & Kane, R. L. (2014). Decision aids for advance care planning: An overview of the state of the science. *Annals of Internal Medicine*, *161*(6), 408–418. https://doi.org/10.7326/M14-0644.

Carabez, R., & Scott, M. (2016). 'Nurses don't deal with these issues:' Nurses' role in advance care planning for lesbian, gay, bisexual and transgender patients. *Journal of Clinical Nursing*, *25*(23–24), 3707–3715. https://doi.org/10.1111/jocn.13336.

Carr, D. (2011). Racial differences in end-of-life planning: Why don't Blacks and Latinos prepare for the inevitable? *OMEGA – Journal of Death and Dying*, *63*(1), 1–20. https://doi.org/10.2190/OM.63.1.a.

Carr, D. (2012a). Racial and ethnic differences in advance care planning: Identifying subgroup patterns and obstacles. *Journal of Aging and Health*, *24*(6), 923–947. https://doi.org/10.1177/0898264312449185.

Carr, D. (2012b). The social stratification of older adults' preparations for end-of-life health care. *Journal of Health and Social Behavior*, *53*(3), 297–312. https://doi.org/10.1177/0022146512455427.

Carr, D. (2012c). "I don't want to die like that …": The impact of significant others' death quality on advance care planning. *The Gerontologist*, *52*(6), 770–781. https://doi.org/10.1093/geront/gns051.

Carr, D., & Khodyakov, D. (2007a). End-of-life health care planning among young-old adults: An assessment of psychosocial influences. *The Journals of Gerontology: Series B*, *62*(2), S135–S141. https://doi.org/10.1093/geronb/62.2.S135.

Carr, D., & Khodyakov, D. (2007b). Health care proxies: Whom do young old adults choose and why? *Journal of Health and Social Behavior*, *48*(2), 180–194. https://doi.org/10.1177/002214650704800206.

Chan, H. M. (2004). Sharing death and dying: Advance directives, autonomy and the family. *Bioethics*, *18*(2), 87–103. https://doi.org/10.1111/j.1467-8519.2004.00383.x.

Cohen, A. B., Wright, M. S., Cooney, L., & Fried, T. (2015). Guardianship and end-of-life decision making. *Journal of the American Medical Association Internal Medicine*, *175*(10), 1687–1691. https://doi.org/10.1001/jamainternmed.2015.3956.

Conrad, P. (2014). *The medicalization of society*. Johns Hopkins University Press.

Devnani, R., Slaven, J. E., Bosslet, G. T., Montz, K., Inger, L., Burke, E. S., & Torke, A. M. (2017). How surrogates decide: A secondary data analysis of decision-making principles used by the surrogates of hospitalized older adults. *Journal of General Internal Medicine, 32*(12), 1285–1293. https://doi.org/10.1007/s11606-017-4158-z.

Ditto, P. H., Jacobson, J. A., Smucker, W. D., Danks, J. H., & Fagerlin, A. (2006). Context changes choices: A prospective study of the effects of hospitalization on life-sustaining treatment preferences. *Medical Decision Making, 26*(4), 313–322. https://doi.org/10.1177/0272989X06290494.

Doukas, D. J. (2017). Advance care planning: Counseling in the wake of CMS reform. *Archives of Family Medicine and General Practice, 1*(2), 48–53.

Drought, T. S., & Koenig, B. A. (2002). Choice in end-of-life decision making: Researching fact or fiction? *The Gerontologist, 42*(suppl_3), 114–128. https://doi.org/10.1093/geront/42.suppl_3.114.

Eisendrath, S. J., & Jonsen, A. R. (1983). The living will: Help or hindrance? *Journal of the American Medical Association, 249*(15), 2054–2058. https://doi.org/10.1001/jama.1983.03330390058032.

Elder, G. H., Johnson, M. K., & Crosnoe, R. (2003). The emergence and development of life course theory. In J. T. Mortimer & M. J. Shanahan (Eds.), *Handbook of the life course* (pp. 3–19). Springer US. https://doi.org/10.1007/978-0-306-48247-2_1.

Emanuel, E. J., Weinberg, D. S., Gonin, R., Hummel, L. R., & Emanuel, L. L. (1993). How well is the Patient Self-Determination Act working? An early assessment. *The American Journal of Medicine, 95*(6), 619–628. https://doi.org/10.1016/0002-9343(93)90358-V.

Emanuel, L. L., Danis, M., Pearlman, R. A., & Singer, P. A. (1995). Advance Care Planning as a Process: Structuring the Discussions in Practice. *Journal of the American Geriatrics Society, 43*(4), 440–446. https://doi.org/10.1111/j.1532-5415.1995.tb05821.x.

Fagerlin, A., & Schneider, C. E. (2004). Enough: The failure of the living will. *Hastings Center Report, 34*(2), 30–42. https://doi.org/10.2307/3527683.

Fairlie, D. E. (2017). Specific words and experience matter to surrogates when making end of life decisions. *Health Communication, 0*(0), 1–7. https://doi.org/10.1080/10410236.2017.1283560.

Fins, J. J., Maltby, B. S., Friedmann, E., Greene, M. G., Norris, K., Adelman, R., & Byock, I. (2005). Contracts, covenants and advance care planning: An empirical study of the moral obligations of patient and proxy. *Journal of Pain and Symptom Management, 29*(1), 55–68. https://doi.org/10.1016/j.jpainsymman.2004.07.004.

Fredriksen-Goldsen, K. I., Hoy-Ellis, C. P., Goldsen, J., Emlet, C. A., & Hooyman, N. R. (2014). Creating a vision for the future: Key competencies and strategies for culturally competent practice with lesbian, gay, bisexual, and transgender (LGBT) older adults in the health and human services. *Journal of Gerontological Social Work, 57*(2–4), 80–107. https://doi.org/10.1080/01634372.2014.890690.

Fried, T. R., Bullock, K., Iannone, L., & O'Leary, J. R. (2009). Understanding advance care planning as a process of health behavior change. *Journal of the American Geriatrics Society, 57*(9), 1547–1555. https://doi.org/10.1111/j.1532-5415.2009.02396.x.

Fried, T. R., Redding, C. A., Robbins, M. L., Paiva, A., O'Leary, J. R., & Iannone, L. (2010). Stages of change for the component behaviors of advance care planning. *Journal of the American Geriatrics Society, 58*(12), 2329–2336. https://doi.org/10.1111/j.1532-5415.2010.03184.x.

Fried, T. R., Zenoni, M., Iannone, L., O'Leary, J., & Fenton, B. T. (2017). Engagement in advance care planning and surrogates' knowledge of patients' treatment goals. *Journal of the American Geriatrics Society*, *65*(8), 1712–1718. https://doi.org/10.1111/jgs.14858.

Fritch, J., Petronio, S., Helft, P. R., & Torke, A. (2013). Making decisions for hospitalized older adults: Ethical factors considered by family surrogates. *The Journal of Clinical Ethics*, *24*(2), 125–134.

Fromme, E. K., Zive, D., Schmidt, T. A., Cook, J. N. B., & Tolle, S. W. (2014). Association between Physician Orders for Life-Sustaining Treatment for Scope of Treatment and in-hospital death in Oregon. *Journal of the American Geriatrics Society*, *62*(7), 1246–1251. https://doi.org/10.1111/jgs.12889.

Garrido, M. M., Harrington, S. T., & Prigerson, H. G. (2014). End-of-life treatment preferences: A key to reducing ethnic/racial disparities in advance care planning? *Cancer*, *120*(24), 3981–3986. https://doi.org/10.1002/cncr.28970.

Garrido, M. M., Idler, E. L., Leventhal, H., & Carr, D. (2013). Pathways from religion to advance care planning: Beliefs about control over length of life and end-of-life values. *The Gerontologist*, *53*(5), 801–816. https://doi.org/10.1093/geront/gns128.

Harrison, K. L., Adrion, E. R., Ritchie, C. S., Sudore, R. L., & Smith, A. K. (2016). Low completion and disparities in advance care planning activities among older Medicare beneficiaries. *Journal of the American Medical Association Internal Medicine*, *176*(12), 1872–1875. https://doi.org/10.1001/jamainternmed.2016.6751.

Hickman, S. E., Moss, A. H., Steinberg, K. E., Sabatino, C. P., & Vandenbroucke, A. (2017). Proposed POLST replacement creates more problems than it solves. *Journal of the American Medical Directors Association*, *18*(12), 1092–1093. https://doi.org/10.1016/j.jamda.2017.09.024.

Hickman, S. E., Nelson, C. A., Perrin, N. A., Moss, A. H., Hammes, B. J., & Tolle, S. W. (2010). A comparison of methods to communicate treatment preferences in nursing facilities: Traditional practices versus the Physician Orders for Life-Sustaining Treatment program. *Journal of the American Geriatrics Society*, *58*(7), 1241–1248. https://doi.org/10.1111/j.1532-5415.2010.02955.x.

Ho, A. (2008). Relational autonomy or undue pressure? Family's role in medical decision-making. *Scandinavian Journal of Caring Sciences*, *22*(1), 128–135. https://doi.org/10.1111/j.1471-6712.2007.00561.x.

Hunter, N. (2010). Rights talk and patient subjectivity: The role of autonomy, equality and participation norms. *Georgetown Law Faculty Publications and Other Works*, 473.

Ikonomidis, S., & Singer, P. A. (1999). Autonomy, liberalism and advance care planning. *Journal of Medical Ethics*, *25*(6), 522–527. https://doi.org/10.1136/jme.25.6.522.

Johnson, K. S., Kuchibhatla, M., & Tulsky, J. A. (2008). What explains racial differences in the use of advance directives and attitudes toward hospice care? *Journal of the American Geriatrics Society*, *56*(10), 1953–1958. https://doi.org/10.1111/j.1532-5415.2008.01919.x.

Kale, M. S., Ornstein, K. A., Smith, C. B., & Kelley, A. S. (2016). End-of-life discussions with older adults. *Journal of the American Geriatrics Society*, *64*(10), 1962–1967. https://doi.org/10.1111/jgs.14285.

Karp, N., & Sabatino, C. (2011). *Improving advanced illness care: The evolution of state POLST programs*. AARP. www.aarp.org/health/doctors-hospitals/info-04-2011/polst-04-11.html.

Kcomt, L., & Gorey, K. M. (2017). End-of-life preparations among lesbian, gay, bisexual, and transgender people: Integrative review of prevalent behaviors. *Journal of Social Work in End-of-Life & Palliative Care*, *13*(4), 284–301. https://doi.org/10.1080/15524256.2017.1387214.

Kelley, A. S., Wenger, N. S., & Sarkisian, C. A. (2010). Opiniones: End-of-life care preferences and planning of older Latinos. *Journal of the American Geriatrics Society*, *58*(6), 1109–1116. https://doi.org/10.1111/j.1532-5415.2010.02853.x.

Kelly, B., Rid, A., & Wendler, D. (2012). Systematic review: Individuals' goals for surrogate decision-making. *Journal of the American Geriatrics Society*, *60*(5), 884–895. https://doi.org/10.1111/j.1532-5415.2012.03937.x.

Khandelwal, N., Kross, E. K., Engelberg, R. A., Coe, N. B., Long, A. C., & Curtis, J. R. (2015). Estimating the effect of palliative care interventions and advance care planning on ICU utilization: A systematic review. *Critical Care Medicine*, *43*(5), 1102–1111. https://doi.org/10.1097/CCM.0000000000000852.

Kim, H.-J., Jen, S., & Fredriksen-Goldsen, K. I. (2017). Race/ethnicity and health-related quality of life among LGBT older adults. *The Gerontologist*, *57*(suppl_1), S30–S39. https://doi.org/10.1093/geront/gnw172.

Kirchhoff, K. T., Hammes, B. J., Kehl, K. A., Briggs, L. A., & Brown, R. L. (2012). Effect of a Disease-Specific Advance Care Planning Intervention on End-of-Life Care. *Journal of the American Geriatrics Society*, *60*(5), 946–950. https://doi.org/10.1111/j.1532-5415.2012.03917.x.

Kong, J., & Moorman, S. M. (2015). Caring for my abuser: Childhood maltreatment and caregiver depression. *The Gerontologist*, *55*(4), 656–666. https://doi.org/10.1093/geront/gnt136.

Koss, C. S., & Baker, T. A. (2017). Race differences in advance directive completion: The narrowing gap between White and African American older adults. *Journal of Aging and Health*, *29*(2), 324–342. https://doi.org/10.1177/0898264316635568.

Kutner, L. (1968). Due process of euthanasia: The living will, a proposal comment. *Indiana Law Journal*, *44*, 539–554.

Kwak, J., & Haley, W. E. (2005). Current research findings on end-of-life decision making among racially or ethnically diverse groups. *The Gerontologist*, *45*(5), 634–641. https://doi.org/10.1093/geront/45.5.634.

Lilley, E. J., Morris, M. A., Sadovnikoff, N., Luxford, J. M., Changoor, N. R., Bystricky, A., Bader, A. M., & Cooper, Z. (2017). "Taking over somebody's life:" Experiences of surrogate decision-makers in the surgical intensive care unit. *Surgery*, *162*(2), 453–460. https://doi.org/10.1016/j.surg.2017.03.011.

Loewenstein, G. (2005). Projection bias in medical decision making. *Medical Decision Making*, *25*(1), 96–105. https://doi.org/10.1177/0272989X04273799.

Loewy, E. H. (2005). In defense of paternalism. *Theoretical Medicine and Bioethics*, *26*(6), 445–468. https://doi.org/10.1007/s11017-005-2203-0.

Lynn, J., Arkes, H. R., Stevens, M., Cohn, F., Koenig, B., Fox, E., Dawson, N. V., Phillips, R. S., Hamel, M. B., & Tsevat, J. (2000). Rethinking fundamental assumptions: SUPPORT'S implications for future reform. *Journal of the American Geriatrics Society*, *48*(S1), S214–S221. https://doi.org/10.1111/j.1532-5415.2000.tb03135.x.

Mack, J. W., Weeks, J. C., Wright, A. A., Block, S. D., & Prigerson, H. G. (2010). End-of-life discussions, goal attainment, and distress at the end of life: Predictors and outcomes of receipt of care consistent with preferences. *Journal of Clinical Oncology*, *28*(7), 1203–1208. https://doi.org/10.1200/JCO.2009.25.4672.

Maioni, A. (1998). *Parting at the crossroads: The emergence of health insurance in the United States and Canada*. Princeton University Press.

Marsack, J., & Stephenson, R. (2017). Exploring the utilization of end-of-life documentation among an online sample of sexual- and gender-minority individuals in the United States. *Journal of Gay & Lesbian Social Services*, *29*(3), 273–279. https://doi.org/10.1080/10538720.2017.1320254.

McPherson, C. J., Wilson, K. G., & Murray, M. A. (2007a). Feeling like a burden: Exploring the perspectives of patients at the end of life. *Social Science & Medicine*, *64*(2), 417–427. https://doi.org/10.1016/j.socscimed.2006.09.013.

McPherson, C. J., Wilson, K. G., & Murray, M. A. (2007b). Feeling like a burden to others: A systematic review focusing on the end of life. *Palliative Medicine*, *21*(2), 115–128. https://doi.org/10.1177/0269216307076345.

Moore, K. A., Rubin, E. B., & Halpern, S. D. (2016). The problems with Physician Orders for Life-Sustaining Treatment. *Journal of the American Medical Association*, *315*(3), 259–260. https://doi.org/10.1001/jama.2015.17362.

Moorman, S. M. (2011a). Older adults' preferences for independent or delegated end-of-life medical decision making. *Journal of Aging and Health*, *23*(1), 135–157. https://doi.org/10.1177/0898264310385114.

Moorman, S. M. (2011b). The importance of feeling understood in marital conversations about end-of-life health care. *Journal of Social and Personal Relationships*, *28*(1), 100–116. https://doi.org/10.1177/0265407510386137.

Moorman, S. M., & Boerner, K. (2018). How social network size and quality affect end-of-life surrogate preferences. *The Journals of Gerontology: Series B*. https://doi.org/10.1093/geronb/gbx031.

Moorman, S. M., & Carr, D. (2008). Spouses' effectiveness as end-of-life health care surrogates: Accuracy, uncertainty, and errors of overtreatment or undertreatment. *The Gerontologist*, *48*(6), 811–819. https://doi.org/10.1093/geront/48.6.811.

Moorman, S. M., & Inoue, M. (2013). Predicting a partner's end-of-life preferences, or substituting one's own? *Journal of Marriage and Family*, *75*(3), 734–745. https://doi.org/10.1111/jomf.12030.

National POLST Paradigm. (2019). *What is POLST?* http://polst.org/.

Nauck, F., Becker, M., King, C., Radbruch, L., Voltz, R., & Jaspers, B. (2014). To what extent are the wishes of a signatory reflected in their advance directive: A qualitative analysis. *BMC Medical Ethics*, *15*, 52. https://doi.org/10.1186/1472-6939-15-52.

Office of Disease Prevention and Health Promotion. (2019). *Lesbian, gay, bisexual, and transgender health*. Healthy People 2020. www.healthypeople.gov/2020/topics-objectives/topic/lesbian-gay-bisexual-and-transgender-health.

Olick, R. S. (2012). Defining features of advance directives in law and clinical practice. *Chest*, *141*(1), 232–238. Scopus. https://doi.org/10.1378/chest.11-1520.

Parks, S. M., Winter, L., Santana, A. J., Parker, B., Diamond, J. J., Rose, M., & Myers, R. E. (2011). Family factors in end-of-life decision-making: Family conflict and proxy relationship. *Journal of Palliative Medicine*, *14*(2), 179–184. https://doi.org/10.1089/jpm.2010.0353.

Pope, T. M. (2012). Legal fundamentals of surrogate decision making. *Chest*, *141*(4), 1074–1081. https://doi.org/10.1378/chest.11-2336.

Portanova, J., Ailshire, J., Rahman, A., & Enguidanos, S. (2017). Ethnic differences in advance directive completion and care preferences: What has changed in a decade? *Journal of the American Geriatrics Society*, *65*(6), 1352–1357. https://doi.org/10.1111/jgs.14800.

Porter, K. E., & Krinsky, L. (2014). Do LGBT aging trainings effectuate positive change in mainstream elder service providers? *Journal of Homosexuality*, *61*(1), 197–216. https://doi.org/10.1080/00918369.2013.835618.

Pruchno, R. A., Rovine, M. J., Cartwright, F., & Wilson-Genderson, M. (2008). Stability and change in patient preferences and spouse substituted judgments regarding dialysis continuation. *The Journals of Gerontology: Series B*, *63*(2), S81–S91. https://doi.org/10.1093/geronb/63.2.S81.

Quill, T. E. (2005). Terri Schiavo – A tragedy compounded. *New England Journal of Medicine, 352*(16), 1630–1633. https://doi.org/10.1056/NEJMp058062.

Randall, F., & Downie, R. S. (2006). *The philosophy of palliative care: Critique and reconstruction.* Oxford University Press.

Raymont, V., Bingley, W., Buchanan, A., David, A. S., Hayward, P., Wessely, S., & Hotopf, M. (2004). Prevalence of mental incapacity in medical inpatients and associated risk factors: Cross-sectional study. *The Lancet, 364*(9443), 1421–1427. https://doi.org/10.1016/S0140-6736(04)17224-3.

SAGE Advocacy and Services for LGBT Elders. (2019). *National resource center on LGBT aging.* LGBTAgingCenter.Org. www.lgbtagingcenter.org/.

Schenker, Y., Crowley-Matoka, M., Dohan, D., Tiver, G. A., Arnold, R. M., & White, D. B. (2012). I don't want to be the one saying 'We should just let him die:' Intrapersonal tensions experienced by surrogate decision makers in the ICU. *Journal of General Internal Medicine, 27*(12), 1657–1665. https://doi.org/10.1007/s11606-012-2129-y.

Schickedanz, A. D., Schillinger, D., Landefeld, C. S., Knight, S. J., Williams, B. A., & Sudore, R. L. (2009). A clinical framework for improving the advance care planning process: Start with patients' self-identified barriers. *Journal of the American Geriatrics Society, 57*(1), 31–39. https://doi.org/10.1111/j.1532-5415.2008.02093.x.

Shalowitz, D. I., Garrett-Mayer, E., & Wendler, D. (2006). The accuracy of surrogate decision makers: A systematic review. *Archives of Internal Medicine, 166*(5), 493–497. https://doi.org/10.1001/archinte.166.5.493.

Shapiro, S. P. (2015). Do advance directives direct? *Journal of Health Politics, Policy and Law, 40*(3), 487–530. https://doi.org/10.1215/03616878-2888424.

Shen, M. J., Prigerson, H. G., Paulk, E., Trevino, K. M., Penedo, F. J., Tergas, A. I., Epstein, A. S., Neugut, A. I., & Maciejewski, P. K. (2016). Impact of end-of-life discussions on the reduction of Latino/non-Latino disparities in do-not-resuscitate order completion. *Cancer, 122*(11), 1749–1756. https://doi.org/10.1002/cncr.29973.

Silveira, M. J., Kim, S. Y. H., & Langa, K. M. (2010). Advance directives and outcomes of surrogate decision making before death. *New England Journal of Medicine, 362*(13), 1211–1218. https://doi.org/10.1056/NEJMsa0907901.

Silveira, M. J., Wiitala, W., & Piette, J. (2014). Advance directive completion by elderly Americans: A decade of change. *Journal of the American Geriatrics Society, 62*(4), 706–710. https://doi.org/10.1111/jgs.12736.

Song, M.-K., Ward, S. E., Fine, J. P., Hanson, L. C., Lin, F.-C., Hladik, G. A., Hamilton, J. B., & Bridgman, J. C. (2015). Advance care planning and end-of-life decision making in dialysis: A randomized controlled trial targeting patients and their surrogates. *American Journal of Kidney Diseases, 66*(5), 813–822. https://doi.org/10.1053/j.ajkd.2015.05.018.

Steinhauser, K. E., Christakis, N. A., Clipp, E. C., McNeilly, M., McIntyre, L., & Tulsky, J. A. (2000). Factors considered important at the end of life by patients, family, physicians, and other care providers. *Journal of the American Medical Association, 284*(19), 2476–2482. https://doi.org/10.1001/jama.284.19.2476.

Stonestreet, E. L. (2014). Love as a regulative ideal in surrogate decision making. *The Journal of Medicine and Philosophy, 39*(5), 523–542. https://doi.org/10.1093/jmp/jhu034.

Stuart, R. B., & Thielke, S. (2017). Standardizing protection of patients' rights from POLST to MOELI (Medical Orders for End-of-Life Intervention). *Journal of the American Medical Directors Association, 18*(9), 741–745. https://doi.org/10.1016/j.jamda.2017.04.022.

Stuart, R. B., & Thielke, S. (2018). Ethical and practical ways in which MOELI (Medical Orders for End-of-Life Intervention) advance the Physician Orders for Life-Sustaining

Treatment (POLST) program. *Journal of the American Medical Directors Association, 19*(3), 270–272. https://doi.org/10.1016/j.jamda.2017.12.004.

Sudore, R. L. (2010). Redefining the "planning" in advance care planning: Preparing for end-of-life decision making. *Annals of Internal Medicine, 153*(4), 256. https://doi.org/10.7326/0003-4819-153-4-201008170-00008.

Sulmasy, D. P., & Snyder, L. (2010). Substituted interests and best judgments: An integrated model of surrogate decision making. *Journal of the American Medical Association, 304*(17), 1946–1947. https://doi.org/10.1001/jama.2010.1595.

Sun, A., Bui, Q., Tsoh, J. Y., Gildengorin, G., Chan, J., Cheng, J., Lai, K., McPhee, S., & Nguyen, T. (2017). Efficacy of a church-based, culturally tailored program to promote completion of advance directives among Asian Americans. *Journal of Immigrant and Minority Health, 19*(2), 381–391. https://doi.org/10.1007/s10903-016-0365-7.

Teno, J. M., Branco, K. J., Mor, V., Phillips, C. D., Hawes, C., Morris, J., & Fries, B. E. (1997). Changes in advance care planning in nursing homes before and after the Patient Self-Determination Act: Report of a 10-state survey. *Journal of the American Geriatrics Society, 45*(8), 939–944. https://doi.org/10.1111/j.1532-5415.1997.tb02963.x.

Teno, J. M., Gruneir, A., Schwartz, Z., Nanda, A., & Wetle, T. (2007). Association between advance directives and quality of end-of-life care: A national study. *Journal of the American Geriatrics Society, 55*(2), 189–194. https://doi.org/10.1111/j.1532-5415.2007.01045.x.

Teno, J. M., Mitchell, S. L., Kuo, S. K., Gozalo, P. L., Rhodes, R. L., Lima, J. C., & Mor, V. (2011). Decision-making and outcomes of feeding tube insertion: A five-state study. *Journal of the American Geriatrics Society, 59*(5), 881–886. https://doi.org/10.1111/j.1532-5415.2011.03385.x.

Terry, P. B., Vettese, M., Song, J., Forman, J., Haller, K. B., Miller, D. J., Stallings, R., & Sulmasy, D. P. (1999). End-of-Life Decision Making: When Patients and Surrogates Disagree. *Journal of Clinical Ethics, 10*(4), 286–293.

Thomeer, M. B., Donnelly, R., Reczek, C., & Umberson, D. (2017). Planning for future care and the end of life: A qualitative analysis of gay, lesbian, and heterosexual couples. *Journal of Health and Social Behavior, 58*(4), 473–487. https://doi.org/10.1177/0022146517735524.

Tinetti, M. E. (2012). The retreat from advanced care planning. *Journal of the American Medical Association, 307*(9), 915–916. https://doi.org/10.1001/jama.2012.229.

Tonelli, M. R. (1996). Pulling the plug on living wills. A critical analysis of advance directives. *Chest, 110*(3), 816–822.

Torke, A. M., Alexander, G. C., & Lantos, J. (2008). Substituted judgment: The limitations of autonomy in surrogate decision making. *Journal of General Internal Medicine, 23*(9), 1514–1517. https://doi.org/10.1007/s11606-008-0688-8.

Torke, A. M., Moloney, R., Siegler, M., Abalos, A., & Alexander, G. C. (2010). Physicians' views on the importance of patient preferences in surrogate decision-making. *Journal of the American Geriatrics Society, 58*(3), 533–538. https://doi.org/10.1111/j.1532-5415.2010.02720.x.

True, G., Phipps, E. J., Braitman, L. E., Harralson, T., Harris, D., & Tester, W. (2005). Treatment preferences and advance care planning at end of life: The role of ethnicity and spiritual coping in cancer patients. *Annals of Behavioral Medicine, 30*(2), 174–179. https://doi.org/10.1207/s15324796abm3002_10.

Vig, E. K., Starks, H., Taylor, J. S., Hopley, E. K., & Fryer-Edwards, K. (2007). Surviving surrogate decision-making: What helps and hampers the experience of making medical decisions for others. *Journal of General Internal Medicine, 22*(9), 1274–1279. https://doi.org/10.1007/s11606-007-0252-y.

Vig, E. K., Taylor, J. S., Starks, H., Hopley, E. K., & Fryer-Edwards, K. (2006). Beyond substituted judgment: How surrogates navigate end-of-life decision-making. *Journal of the American Geriatrics Society*, *54*(11), 1688–1693. https://doi.org/10.1111/j.1532-5415.2006.00911.x.

Wahlert, L., & Fiester, A. (2013). A false sense of security: Lesbian, gay, bisexual, and transgender (LGBT) surrogate health care decision-making rights. *The Journal of the American Board of Family Medicine*, *26*(6), 802–804. https://doi.org/10.3122/jabfm.2013.06.130130.

Weiss, B. D., Berman, E. A., Howe, C. L., & Fleming, R. B. (2012). Medical decision-making for older adults without family. *Journal of the American Geriatrics Society*, *60*(11), 2144–2150. https://doi.org/10.1111/j.1532-5415.2012.04212.x.

Wendler, D., & Rid, A. (2011). Systematic review: The effect on surrogates of making treatment decisions for others. *Annals of Internal Medicine*, *154*(5), 336. https://doi.org/10.7326/0003-4819-154-5-201103010-00008.

Will, J. F. (2011a). A brief historical and theoretical perspective on patient autonomy and medical decision making: Part I: The beneficence model. *Chest*, *139*(3), 669–673. Scopus. https://doi.org/10.1378/chest.10-2532.

Will, J. F. (2011b). A brief historical and theoretical perspective on patient autonomy and medical decision making: Part II: The autonomy model. *Chest*, *139*(6), 1491–1497. Scopus. https://doi.org/10.1378/chest.11-0516.

Winter, L. (2013). Patient values and preferences for end-of-life treatments: Are values better predictors than a living will? *Journal of Palliative Medicine*, *16*(4), 362–368. https://doi.org/10.1089/jpm.2012.0303.

Winter, L., Moss, M. S., & Hoffman, C. (2009). Affective forecasting and advance care planning: Anticipating quality of life in future health statuses. *Journal of Health Psychology*, *14*(3), 447–456. https://doi.org/10.1177/1359105309102201.

Winter, L., & Parks, S. M. (2012a). The reluctance to burden others as a value in end-of-life decision making: A source of inaccuracy in substituted judgment. *Journal of Health Psychology*, *17*(2), 179–188. https://doi.org/10.1177/1359105311414956.

Winter, L., & Parks, S. M. (2012b). Acceptors and rejecters of life-sustaining treatment: Differences in advance care planning characteristics. *Journal of Applied Gerontology*, *31*(6), 734–742. https://doi.org/10.1177/0733464811399079.

Wolff, J. L., & Boyd, C. M. (2015). A look at person-centered and family-centered care among older adults: Results from a national survey. *Journal of General Internal Medicine*, *30*(10), 1497–1504. https://doi.org/10.1007/s11606-015-3359-6.

Yadav, K. N., Gabler, N. B., Cooney, E., Kent, S., Kim, J., Herbst, N., Mante, A., Halpern, S. D., & Courtright, K. R. (2017). Approximately one in three U.S. adults completes any type of advance directive for end-of-life care. *Health Affairs*, *36*(7), 1244–1251. https://doi.org/10.1377/hlthaff.2017.0175.

8

EUTHANASIA

The word euthanasia is a broad term that encompasses a number of actions – or inactions – that result in death. Active euthanasia may represent the ultimate in predictable death, with people choosing the time and place of death. With regard to human life, some forms of euthanasia are widely acceptable to lawyers, ethicists, religious leaders, and the general public, while others are much more contentious. In this chapter, I explore some of the medical and ethical questions surrounding euthanasia, and focus on the potential for systemic disparities in its use. This chapter ends with an analysis of racial and ethnic differences in public opinion on forms of euthanasia, with data from the 2013 Pew Research Center's Religion and Public Life Project.

Passive Euthanasia

Terminology is important in discussions of euthanasia. Euthanasia can be passive or active, where passive refers to permitting death, or doing nothing to prevent it, while active refers to taking action to cause death. Either passive or active euthanasia can be voluntary, non-voluntary, or involuntary. Voluntary has its usual meaning of *chosen*, while in the terminology of bioethics, involuntary and non-voluntary are not synonymous. The term non-voluntary is reserved for conditions in which the patient is unable to either consent or refuse, while the term involuntary refers to actions that occur despite the patient's explicit refusal of consent. Table 8.1 illustrates a classification of types of euthanasia according to whether they are passive or active and whether they are voluntary, non-voluntary, or involuntary, with select examples from the chapter.

Law in the U.S. recognizes the right of an adult patient who has decision-making capacity to refuse treatment, including life-saving or life-sustaining treatment

TABLE 8.1 Classification of Types of Euthanasia, with Examples

	Voluntary	*Non-Voluntary (Patient cannot consent)*	*Involuntary (Patient refuses consent)*
Passive	Do-not-resuscitate order	Withdrawing life-sustaining treatment for an incapacitated person	Hospital withdraws treatment against patient/family wishes
Active	Physician-assisted death	Groningen Protocol (Netherlands)	Murder

(Cooper, 2010). This choice is voluntary passive euthanasia. Most people who complete advance care plans, such as living wills, do so to request passive euthanasia (Winter & Parks, 2012). For example, a patient who has a do-not-resuscitate order is making a request for passive euthanasia. Patients and families who decide to discontinue treatment with artificial nutrition or hydration, a ventilator, or other equipment or medication that is sustaining life are also choosing passive euthanasia.

The United States Supreme Court has affirmed the right to die, even when ending treatment is non-voluntary. For example, Terri Schiavo was a young woman who, following a heart attack, was in a persistent vegetative state for 15 years (Clark, 2005). Her husband wished to remove her feeding tube and allow her to die, while her parents wished to continue artificial nutrition. Following a seven-year court battle, Schiavo's feeding tube was removed and she died in 2005. In a non-voluntary case such as Schiavo's, health care professionals and family are legally able to choose passive euthanasia if all agree that it is in the best interests of the patient (Quill, 2005). Decisions are litigated only when stakeholders, such as two sides of a family, disagree about what is best for the patient.

However, the Supreme Court has stopped short of declaring passive euthanasia to be a fundamental or absolute right, having recognized cases in which the state can compel a person to receive treatment. For example, in 1982, the parents of a baby born with Down's syndrome, called Baby Doe in the judicial record, elected not to treat the baby's fistula although it was medically correctable (Caplan et al., 2012). The baby died six days after birth, and subsequently federal child abuse laws were amended to require life-prolonging treatment in such cases. Although some ethicists have argued that this particular legal case made a poor basis for a law that applies to all children born with disabilities, the law often compels U.S. pediatricians to provide infants with life-prolonging care even if their prognosis is extremely poor (Caplan et al., 2012; Kopelman, 2005).

Finally, involuntary passive euthanasia occurs if health care professionals withhold or withdraw treatment against the wishes of a patient or the patient's legally recognized surrogate. For example, baby Tinslee Lewis was born prematurely, and physicians have concluded that she has no hope of survival and that life-prolonging treatment causes her to suffer (Iait, 2020; Zraick, 2020). That is, allowing Tinslee to die is in her best interests because further treatment would be futile: It would not help, and could even harm, her (Nair-Collins, 2017). However, her family is suing to continue treatment. This case is ongoing at the time of publication, but in similar cases, the law has sided with medical professionals (Pope, 2008). Cases like Terri Schiavo, Baby Doe, and Tinslee Lewis illustrate the tragic situations that can arise around deaths that are not predictable, but rather are now-rare occurrences involving young people.

Active Euthanasia

However, what most members of the public think of when they hear the word *euthanasia* is not withholding or withdrawing treatment, but rather taking some action to hasten death, or active euthanasia. Broadly speaking, active involuntary euthanasia is murder: The murderer engages in an action designed to kill the victim against the victim's wishes and without the victim's consent. Active involuntary euthanasia is illegal in all jurisdictions.

Active non-voluntary euthanasia is also illegal in all jurisdictions, and it is tacitly permitted in only one. The Groningen Protocol is a practice in the Netherlands that describes situations in which a physician may actively euthanize a newborn who is unbearably and incurably suffering (Verhagen & Sauer, 2005a, 2005b). The parents must initiate the request and consent to it. Even so, the practice is not legal in the Netherlands; rather, there is simply a reluctance to prosecute physicians who have adhered to the Protocol. The Protocol has been used extremely rarely, on perhaps only two infants in the five years between 2005 and 2010 (Verhagen, 2014). Many ethicists object to the Protocol, and there are no similar cases anywhere else in the world (Chervenak et al., 2006; Jotkowitz & Glick, 2006; Jotkowitz et al., 2008). A surrogate decision-maker in the U.S. cannot choose active death for an incapacitated person of any age, and a physician certainly cannot perform it.

Forms of voluntary active euthanasia are much more open for debate in the U.S. and around the world. One form of voluntary active euthanasia is suicide, or ending one's own life. Since 1977, the General Social Survey (GSS) has been asking the U.S. public the question "Do you think a person has a right to end his or her own life if this person has an incurable disease?" and increasingly, the public says yes (Duncan & Parmelee, 2006). In 1977, 38% of GSS respondents approved, and in 2014, 60% of respondents approved (Attell, 2015). Accordingly, the debate around the rationality of suicide has changed. Suicide prevention continues to be a major topic in psychiatry and public health (Zalsman et al., 2016), but increasingly, the mainstream views suicide in the face of terminal illness as a sensible and valid choice (Barry, 2017; Werth Jr., 1996). For example, early diagnosis of Alzheimer's disease has greatly advanced, but there remains no cure. One argument reasons that health care professionals have a duty to reveal such a diagnosis to patients, so that patients may choose to pre-empt their suffering through suicide (Davis, 2014).

Alongside the change in public opinion about suicide, the suicide rate in the United States has been increasing. In 2017, the U.S. recorded the highest suicide rate since 1942, which was a 33% increase since 1999 (Hedegaard et al., 2018). Suicide increased most sharply in rural areas, alongside the rate of fatal opioid overdoses (Peters et al., 2019). Researchers have labeled such deaths, which are concentrated among non-Hispanic Whites with low-educational attainment in midlife, *deaths of despair* (Stein et al., 2017). The media has even begun to cover the tragic group of parents who have lost more than one adult child to drug overdose (Dwyer, 2019). Deaths of despair seems quite different from the predictable death, which occurs in older adulthood from chronic disease. Deaths of despair are regionally concentrated in places that have experienced stagnant or declining life expectancy since 1980 (Bor, 2017; Monnat et al., 2019). Of course, deaths of despair contribute to life expectancy figures, but researchers believe that these deaths are the result of the economic marginalization of people with low levels of education who live in parts of the country once known for manufacturing and production (Cherlin, 2018).

The sharp increase in suicide deaths is especially striking given that statisticians estimate that perhaps over 90% of suicide attempts fail (National Institute of Mental Health, 2019). Dying by suicide is not readily achievable, and the means of suicide commonly available to most people are violent, prolonged, or painful. Patients who are suffering from terminal illnesses may wish to die but be too disabled to be able to carry out suicide. Thus, individuals the world over seek help from health care professionals to engage in voluntary active euthanasia. As of 2019, a physician could legally euthanize an adult patient under some conditions in five countries: Belgium, Canada, Colombia, Luxembourg, and the Netherlands. The Netherlands permits children as young as 12 to select to have a physician perform voluntary active euthanasia, and in 2014, the practice became legal for minors in Belgium, again under certain conditions (Dan et al., 2014; Siegel et al., 2014). Conditions for both adults and children include confirmation of unbearable suffering, the patient's legal competence, and so on.

In most parts of the world, however, the state has balked at the concept of permitting a health care professional, whose duty is to heal, to end a human life. Voluntary active euthanasia by a physician is against the code of medical ethics espoused by many professional organizations of health care providers, including the American Medical Association (American Medical Association, 2019). The title of a 2011 physician commentary, "Can you even imagine teaching medical students how to end their patients' lives?" perhaps best encapsulates this viewpoint (Boudreau, 2011). There are also concerns about physicians' ability to judge who is suffering unbearably and who is not, as well as concerns about terminally ill persons being coerced into euthanasia (Keown, 2018; Sulmasy, Travaline, et al., 2016). Of course, in addition to these secular arguments, there are also moral objections rooted in various religious faith traditions.

Some ethicists draw a distinction between active voluntary euthanasia by a physician, the act of ending a patient's life, and physician-assisted death (PAD), the act of providing a patient with the means to end his or her own life.[1] Famously, U.S. physician Jack Kevorkian spent 8 years in prison for second degree murder for his 1998 lethal injection of a consenting, terminally-ill adult patient (Charatan, 1999). In comparison, PAD involves a doctor writing a prescription for a lethal dose of a drug, and then the patient may fill the prescription and self-administer the drug. The debate about active voluntary euthanasia by a physician vs. PAD is far from settled, with some bioethicists arguing that there are few, if any, meaningful distinctions between the two acts (Dixon, 1998; Sulmasy, Ely, et al., 2016). Nevertheless, PAD has gained legal traction in the U.S., particularly following the 2014 death of 30-year-old Brittany Maynard, a brain cancer patient who became an outspoken advocate for PAD (Gostin & Roberts, 2016). As of 2020, PAD was legal in a wider array of places than active voluntary euthanasia by a physician was, including the U.S. states of California, Colorado, Hawaii, Maine, Montana, New Jersey, Oregon, Vermont, and Washington, as well as in the District of Colombia. In all of these jurisdictions, PAD is available only to legally competent, terminally ill adults who have completed a strict protocol. For example, Table 8.2 lists the process that doctors and patients are required to follow under Oregon's Death with Dignity Act.

TABLE 8.2 Legal Process of Physician-Assisted Death in Oregon

1	The patient makes an initial verbal request for PAD to their physician.
2	15-day waiting period.
3	The patient makes a second verbal request for PAD.
4	The patient completes a form requesting PAD. The form is signed by the patient and two witnesses, at least one of whom must *not* be: ❑ a relative of the patient; ❑ an heir of the patient; or ❑ an employee of a health care facility where the patient receives treatment.
5	48-hour waiting period.
6	Physician may write a prescription, and has one week to file confirmation with the state that: ❑ the patient is an Oregon resident who has a terminal illness and less than 6 months to live; ❑ a second physician has confirmed the diagnosis and prognosis; ❑ the patient does not have impaired judgment due to a psychiatric or psychological disorder, including depression; and ❑ the patient has been fully informed at least twice about their condition, the risks of PAD, and alternatives to PAD.
7	A pharmacy dispenses the prescription and within 10 days, reports the dispensation to the state.
8	Within 10 days of the patient's death, the physician files a form with the state explaining cause of death. If PAD was the cause, the physician reports who attended the death, where it occurred, how long it took, and whether there were complications.

From Oregon Health Authority, 2020.

Oregon began to permit PAD in 1997, and so there are over 20 years of data on the practice. In the first 20 years of the law, 374 physicians wrote prescriptions for a lethal dose of medication for 1,857 people (Blanke et al., 2017; Hedberg & New, 2017). Interestingly, of the 1,857 people who received a prescription, only 64% filled the prescription and consumed the drug. Nearly 80% of decedents had cancer. Over 600,000 people died in the state during the 20-year period, meaning that physician-assisted deaths accounted for less than 0.25% of deaths.

Washington State began allowing PAD in 2008, and like Oregon, issues reports annually (Washington State Department of Health, 2019). There, 115 physicians wrote prescriptions for 212 patients in 2017, and 164 of those (77%) died from taking the medication. Similar to Oregon, 72% had cancer. The typical patient died at home less than 90 minutes after taking the drug, with a health care provider – though rarely the prescribing physician – present.

Indirect Euthanasia

Indirect euthanasia is a practice that does not fall neatly into the passive/active and voluntary/non-voluntary/involuntary classification scheme. One definition is "allowing death to occur without a direct link between the action, intent, and result" (Terry, 1995 p. 189). Death is among the known side effects of the treatment, but is not the goal of the treatment. That is, some medical treatments ease extreme suffering but also hasten death.

In practice, however, there is little clarity about what treatments constitute indirect euthanasia. Palliative sedation therapy, or "the use of sedative medication to relieve intolerable and refractory distress by reducing patient consciousness," (Morita et al., 2002, p. 447) was first reported in the medical literature in 1990 (Ventafridda et al., 1990). Sedative medications relieve symptoms such as delirium and labored breathing, but sufficient quantities will stop the heart and lungs, and so palliative sedation may be a form of indirect euthanasia.

However, referring to palliative sedation therapy as a single practice is a misnomer, since there is wide variation in "degree of sedation, duration, pharmacological properties of medications, target symptoms, and target patients" (Morita et al., 2002, p. 451). Several meta-analytic studies have documented forms of palliative sedation that do not hasten death (Maeda et al., 2016; Maltoni et al., 2012). In 2010, 10% of a random sample of practicing U.S. physicians said they had practiced palliative sedation, and they held disparate opinions about whether and when it was an acceptable practice (Putman et al., 2013). Most agree that palliative sedation is an acceptable treatment of last resort, but they vary on how deeply sedated the patient should be, how long such treatment should be used, what kinds of symptoms merit sedation, whether artificial nutrition and hydration should accompany sedation, and which sedatives should be used (Gurschick et al., 2015; Schildmann & Schildmann, 2014). In particular, opinions vary over whether palliative sedation is appropriate for handling psychosocial or existential suffering in addition to physical suffering (Lam et al., 2017; Rodrigues et al., 2018).

Palliative sedation is legal everywhere in the United States (Ollove, 2018), but because of these definitional issues, especially concerning physicians' intent, there are no robust estimates of its prevalence. Estimates from elsewhere in the world tend to be restricted to deaths that occurred in hospital-based palliative care units, or deaths from cancer, or some other small and limited group of decedents. For example, 21% of such deaths in palliative care hospital units in Austria in 2012–2013 involved intermittent or continuous sedation (Schur et al., 2016). Even in countries where voluntary active euthanasia by a physician is legal, physicians may elect to mislabel a euthanasia case as a palliative sedation case so as to avoid social censure or even legal proceedings (Papavasiliou & Payne, 2015).

Social Disparities in Euthanasia

There are two prevalent concerns regarding social inequalities and euthanasia in the U.S., one stemming from proponents of physician involvement and one stemming from opponents of physician involvement. Those in favor worry that privileged people would have preferential access to voluntary active euthanasia by a physician or to PAD, such that marginalized persons would be unable to use these services if they desired them. Meanwhile, those opposed worry that society will begin to rely upon the practices as an expedient means of alleviating social problems, such as mental illness, physical disability, and the cost of improving end-of-life care. In this scenario, marginalized people would be at risk of being coerced into procedures to end their lives prematurely. Physicians' involvement in Nazi genocide as well as the United States's own ugly history with eugenics are raised as cautionary tales (Grodin et al., 2017; Joseph, 2005). Fundamental cause theory would posit that any systematic abuses would disproportionately affect the poor, racial and ethnic minorities, and other disadvantaged groups; therefore, the concerns of both proponents and opponents might be valid.

Concerning the argument that only elites might be able to access assisted death, medical anthropologist Mara Buchbinder conducted an ethnographic study in Vermont between 2015 and 2017, in order to study how the state implemented PAD. She found that the cost of the most common drug doctors prescribed was high, and that most patients did not have insurance coverage for it (Buchbinder, 2018b). Doctors were able to identify alternative drugs, but expressed concern that these other options were not as safe or effective. Doctors also felt that patients who wanted PAD needed to be well informed about law, knowledgeable about medical practices, and persistent in seeking services (Buchbinder, 2018b). Research in other states confirms these findings: In Oregon, people with college degrees were ten times more likely to use PAD than were people who had not completed high school (Hedberg & New, 2017). California passed a law permitting Medicaid to pay for PAD drugs, because the out-of-pocket cost was prohibitive for some patients (Petrillo et al., 2017).

Buchbinder also found that the continued prohibition on voluntary active euthanasia by a physician in Vermont imposed some dependencies upon patients (Buchbinder, 2018a). That is, a health care professional cannot administer the lethal drug, yet almost all patients require some assistance to consume it. Socially isolated people who wanted PAD were thus sometimes unable to have it. However, patients very rarely died alone, which many patients and bereaved persons found deeply reassuring (Buchbinder, 2018a).

At the same time, Buchbinder's work uncovered some of the concerns that opponents of PAD express. Vermont doctors and families were actively debating the physician's role: Should a patient always be the party that raises the topic of PAD, or are there times when a physician can ethically do so? If a physician does present PAD as an option, what language makes the conversation informative rather than advisory (Buchbinder, 2019)?

Then, once a patient had chosen PAD, care providers were "deeply implicated" in the process (Buchbinder et al., 2018 p. 936). They actively assisted the dying person in taking the drug and waited for the person to die, and sometimes felt that their own emotional needs had to be put on hold until after the death. Family and friends who assembled for the death described needing to be brave, and sometimes having to encourage the patient to take the drug at the last moment. Buchbinder uncovered no cases of coercion, but the processes involved were certainly ones that could be perverted by a rushed physician or burned-out care provider.

Perhaps the largest practical concern of those who argue that PAD could become a quick fix is whether palliative care is available and accessible in places where PAD has been legalized (Bélanger et al., 2019). That is, where PAD is practiced, has it replaced high-quality palliative care? Do patients feel pressured into PAD because there are no other ways to realize a comfortable and peaceful death? Thus far, there is little evidence that this problem has occurred (Albaladejo, 2019). Over 20 years in Oregon, 88% of patients who selected PAD were enrolled in hospice (Hedberg & New, 2017). Similarly, in Belgium, decedents who had voluntary active euthanasia by a physician were more likely to have received palliative care services than decedents who did not (Dierickx et al., 2018). In Europe more broadly, access to palliative care has expanded more quickly in nations with legal voluntary active euthanasia by a physician than in countries that do not allow it (Chambaere & Bernheim, 2015). Certainly, both proponents and critics of PAD and other active euthanasia practices will continue to monitor the data on the spread and acceptance of the practices in the U.S. and elsewhere.

Data from the Survey of Aging and Longevity

Race and ethnicity is a key fundamental cause of disparities in the predictable death in the U.S. For example, Black non-Hispanic persons experience the deaths of friends and loved ones more frequently than do White non-Hispanic

Americans (Umberson, 2017; Umberson et al., 2017). Moreover, their deaths are less likely to be peaceful and comfortable: Persons of color are more likely than White non-Hispanic persons to die in the intensive care unit and in the hospital, and less likely to receive hospice services (LoPresti et al., 2016; Tschirhart et al., 2014). Perhaps accordingly, although not all studies find group differences (Periyakoil et al., 2016), race and ethnicity does often contribute to variations in public opinion about forms of euthanasia. For example, focus groups with White non-Hispanic, Black non-Hispanic, or Hispanic Californians yielded different insights (Cain & McCleskey, 2019). Participants of all backgrounds generally approved of the new PAD law in the state, but Black non-Hispanic and Hispanic participants had more nuanced opinions. They raised issues of alleviating suffering and burden, but also issues of religious belief, risks to vulnerable patients, and shortcuts in quality of care.

In the remainder of this chapter, I conduct an analysis of public opinion data on passive and active euthanasia, focusing on similarities and differences across racial and ethnic groups. In 2013, the Pew Research Center surveyed a random sample of the U.S. public about euthanasia as part of the Religion and Public Life Project. Participants included 1,832 men and women who identified as White non-Hispanic, Black non-Hispanic, or Hispanic. Their sociodemographic characteristics are presented in Table 8.3. Additional statistics are available in the Pew Center's own reports on the survey (Pew Research Center, 2013a, 2013b, 2013c). Further technical details about the sample and the study design are available in the Appendix to this chapter; for example, Table 8.A1 includes participants' characteristics by racial or ethnic group.

First, survey respondents answered a question about passive euthanasia for a hypothetical person. They were asked

> Which comes closer to your view? In all circumstances, doctors and nurses should do everything possible to save the life of a patient. Or, sometimes there are circumstances where a patient should be allowed to die.

Sixty-nine percent of participants said that there are circumstances where a patient should be allowed to die, while 31% said that in all circumstances, doctors and nurses should do everything possible to save the life of a patient. There were statistically significant differences by race and ethnicity, however, with non-Hispanic Whites much more likely than the other two groups to endorse the idea that there are circumstances in which a patient should be allowed to die. Among non-Hispanic Whites, 82% thought that there were such circumstances, while only 49% of non-Hispanic Blacks and 43% of Hispanics thought so.

Second, participants answered a series of three questions about their own personal preferences for passive euthanasia. The questions were worded:

TABLE 8.3 Characteristics of Participants, 2013 Pew Research Center Survey on Aging and Longevity, $N = 1{,}832$

	%	*n*
Race/ethnicity		
White non-Hispanic	65	1,189
Black non-Hispanic	18	327
Hispanic	17	316
Female	53	973
Educational attainment		
Less than high school	9	155
High school graduate	26	480
Some college	27	494
BA or more	38	692
Region		
Northeast	14	264
Midwest	17	319
South	46	844
West	22	405
Median income	\$40,000 to \$49,999	–
Foreign-born	12	226
Religious affiliation		
Mainline Protestant	19	347
Evangelical Protestant	31	563
Roman Catholic	23	410
Other affiliation	7	127
Unaffiliated	19	348
Average age in years	51.5 ($SD = 18.2$)	–

> Now I'm going to describe a few medical situations that sometimes happen, and for each one, please tell me what you would want your own doctor to do, if you could make the choice. If you had a disease with no hope of improvement and you were suffering a great deal of physical pain, would you tell your doctor to do everything possible to save your life, or would you tell your doctor to stop treatment so you could die? How about if you had a disease with no hope of improvement that made it hard for you to function in your day-to-day activities? How about if you had an illness that made you totally dependent on a family member or other person for all of your care?

I combined the information from these three questions to create an indicator of whether the respondent would ever want to stop treatment, or whether the respondent would want to continue treatment in all scenarios. Seventy percent of people identified at least one of the three scenarios as one in which they would want their doctor to stop treatment, while 30% said that their doctor should do everything possible to save their life in all three scenarios. Here, each racial or ethnic group was distinctly different, statistically speaking. Seventy-nine percent of White non-Hispanic participants wanted to stop treatment in some scenario, as compared to 63% of Hispanics and 47% of Black non-Hispanics.

Third, participants were asked a series of questions about suicide, without specifying whether it included intervention from another person. The question read,

> Do you think a person has a moral right to end his or her own life under any of the following circumstances?

The four circumstances were "when this person has a disease that is incurable;" "when this person is suffering great pain and has no hope of improvement;" "when this person is an extremely heavy burden on his or her family;" and "when this person is ready to die because living has become a burden." I combined the answers from these four questions to create an indicator of whether the respondent ever or never condoned suicide. Sixty-six percent of participants agreed that suicide was a moral right in at least one of the four conditions, and 34% of participants said that suicide was not a person's moral right, regardless of circumstances. Hispanic and non-Hispanic Whites were about equally likely to agree, at 70 and 68 percent, respectively. Non-Hispanic Blacks were less likely to agree, with 57% saying that people have a moral right to suicide.

Finally, participants indicated their opinion about PAD. The question read,

> In some states, it's legal for doctors to prescribe lethal doses of drugs that a terminally ill patient could use themselves to commit suicide. Do you approve or disapprove of laws that let doctors assist patients who want to end their lives this way?

Forty-seven percent of participants approved, and 53% disapproved. The majority of non-Hispanic Whites, 55%, approved. This figure was significantly larger than the proportions of non-Hispanic Blacks (30%) and Hispanics (36%) who approved.

I noticed that hypothetical passive euthanasia, passive euthanasia for oneself, and moral right to suicide each yielded an approximate 70–30 split between those in favor and those against the form of euthanasia across racial/ethnic groups. I was curious to know whether in each case it was the same people approving and disapproving of the measure. I was also curious to know how opinions about PAD corresponded with opinions about the other three issues. Therefore, Table 8.4 shows a cross-tabulation of participants' answers to the four topics.

Somewhat surprisingly, there were respondents who gave every possible combination of answers. That is, for the first three questions, the group of 30% in opposition to the type of euthanasia was comprised of different participants, and responses on those topics did not determine attitudes towards PAD. The data

TABLE 8.4 Public Opinion on Passive and Active Euthanasia, 2013 Pew Research Center Survey on Aging and Longevity, $N = 1{,}579$

Approve of passive euthanasia for others	*Approve of passive euthanasia for self*	*Moral right to suicide*	*Approve of PAD*	*n*	%
Yes	Yes	Yes	Yes	565	35.8
Yes	Yes	No	No	173	11.0
Yes	Yes	Yes	No	159	10.1
No	No	No	No	159	10.1
No	Yes	Yes	No	80	5.1
No	No	Yes	No	78	4.9
No	Yes	No	No	73	4.6
Yes	No	No	No	69	4.4
Yes	No	Yes	Yes	67	4.2
No	Yes	Yes	Yes	53	3.4
Yes	No	Yes	No	30	1.9
No	No	Yes	Yes	28	1.8
Yes	Yes	No	Yes	16	1.0
No	No	No	Yes	12	0.8
Yes	No	No	Yes	9	0.6
No	Yes	No	Yes	8	0.5

indicate that people have nuanced opinions, attitudes, and beliefs about this complex set of issues concerning life and death.

That said, there were four common patterns of response that each described the views of 10% or more of the sample. Slightly over one-third (35.8%) of respondents approved of all forms of euthanasia. They approved of both passive forms, including limiting treatment for themselves and for a hypothetical other, and they approved of active forms such as suicide and PAD. Eleven percent of participants approved of passive – limiting treatment for self and hypothetical others – but not the active forms of euthanasia. Finally, 10% approved of everything except PAD, involving a doctor in the process of ending one's life. Finally, ten percent opposed all four forms of euthanasia, pursuing the continuation of life in all cases. The remainder of the analysis concerns the 1,056 people in these four larger groups.

The four groups differed in their racial/ethnic composition, as illustrated in Table 8.5. White non-Hispanic people were overrepresented in the group approving of passive euthanasia but opposing active euthanasia and in the group approving of all forms of euthanasia. Both Black non-Hispanic people and Hispanic people were overrepresented in the group opposing all forms of euthanasia and in the group approving of passive euthanasia and suicide, but not PAD.

The statistics presented thus far may be somewhat misleading, insofar as the participants differed in ways other than race and ethnicity. For example, participants in each group ranged in age from 18 to 90, but the average age of non-Hispanic

TABLE 8.5 Racial/Ethnic Composition of the Overall Sample and Four Common Opinions, 2013 Pew Research Center Survey on Aging and Longevity, $N = 1{,}056$

	White non-Hispanic	*Black non-Hispanic*	*Hispanic*
	%	%	%
Overall sample	72	14	13
Oppose passive and active euthanasia	35	26	38
Approve passive, oppose active	83	6	12
Approve passive and suicide, oppose PAD	63	20	18
Approve passive and active euthanasia	82	10	7

Whites was 55 years old, while it was 49 for non-Hispanic Blacks and 43 for Hispanics. These age differences could confound the numbers on racial or ethnic difference, if for example younger people are more permissive towards euthanasia than older people are. Therefore, I conducted regression analyses that allowed me to compare the groups according to their composition on multiple factors simultaneously. I chose as factors many of the aspects of inequality that I cover in this book: race/ethnicity, primarily, and also gender, educational attainment, region of the country, income, and immigrant status. Further, I included religious affiliation, given that it is a focus of the Pew Center's work, and age. I did not include sexual orientation because the Pew survey did not ask participants for this information.

The columns in Table 8.6 show the estimated probability of being in each opinion group for someone who has the characteristic listed in that row, and is average or normative with regard to the other characteristics. For example, the typical White non-Hispanic participant had a 63% chance of approving of all forms of euthanasia. Table 8.A2, in the Appendix, shows the results of the regression analysis in the form of odds ratios, which will be more familiar than predicted probabilities to readers with greater experience in social statistics.

There are large differences based on many of these characteristics, including race or ethnicity. Other factors being equal, people who were White non-Hispanic were most likely to approve of all four forms of euthanasia, at a 63% probability. There was only a 7% chance that a White non-Hispanic participant opposed all four methods. Notably, the average Black non-Hispanic and Hispanic participants were also most likely to approve of all four types of euthanasia, but they were much more evenly divided across the four groups. A Black non-Hispanic participant had a 40% probability of approving of all four methods, and a 31% probability of opposing all four methods, for example. A Hispanic participant had a 49% likelihood of approving of all four methods, and a 25% chance of approving of passive euthanasia and suicide, but not PAD. The main message from this analysis

TABLE 8.6 Multiple Multinomial Logistic Regression of Racial/Ethnic Differences in Attitudes toward Euthanasia, Results Presented as Predicted Probabilities, 2013 Pew Research Center Survey on Aging and Longevity, $N = 1{,}056$

	Oppose passive and active euthanasia	*Approve passive, oppose active*	*Approve passive and suicide, oppose PAD*	*Approve passive and active euthanasia*
Race/ethnicity				
White non-Hispanic	7	16	14	63
Black non-Hispanic	31	9	21	40
Hispanic	18	8	25	49
Gender				
Female	10	15	16	59
Male	10	12	18	60
Educational attainment				
Less than high school	23	6	43	28
High school graduate	15	16	22	47
Some college	10	13	14	62
BA or more	7	13	14	66
Region				
Northeast	9	11	11	69
Midwest	8	18	23	51
South	11	16	17	56
West	9	9	18	64
Income ($40,000–49,999)	14	17	16	54
Country of birth				
U.S.	9	14	17	60
Foreign-born	23	12	17	48
Religious affiliation				
Mainline Protestant	8	10	18	65
Evangelical Protestant	15	34	19	32
Roman Catholic	10	12	18	60
Other affiliation	16	18	10	55
Unaffiliated	4	4	10	82
Age (51.5 years)	14	16	15	55

of race and ethnicity is that persons of color have a wider variety of opinions about euthanasia than do their White non-Hispanic peers.

Other notable findings concerned educational attainment and religious affiliation. The more education a person had, the more likely that he or she supported all four forms of euthanasia. A college graduate had a 66% probability of approving of all four, whereas a person who had not completed high school had only a 28% chance of complete approval. People who had not completed high school were especially likely to oppose PAD. Turning to religious affiliation, Evangelical Protestants stood out for their opposition to euthanasia, especially the active types (i.e., suicide and PAD). People of all other affiliations were most likely to approve of all four questions. Indeed, participants who had no religious affiliation had an 82% chance of approving of all manners of euthanasia.

Combining characteristics shows even more dramatic differences (not tabulated). For example, a White non-Hispanic college graduate who lived in the Northeast, was born in the U.S., and had no religious affiliation had an 93% chance of approving of all four euthanasia questions, and only a 1% chance of disapproving of all four. For comparison, a Hispanic person who had not completed high school, lived in the South, was born abroad, and was an Evangelical Protestant would have only a 4% chance of approving of all four questions, and a 66% chance of disapproving of all four.

Some groups are better represented among lawmakers, and therefore may have a better chance of having their preferences reflected in policy or practice. People of color and people with low levels of educational attainment are poorly represented. The year 2019, for example, ushered in a U.S. Congress well lauded for racial and ethnic diversity, and yet only three of 100 Senators were non-Hispanic Black and an additional four were Hispanic (United States Senate, 2019). Further, in the House of Representatives in the 116th Congress, 72% of members had not only completed college, but also attained a graduate degree (Burgat & Hunt, 2018). Nevertheless, laws are more conservative than a mostly White, well-educated lawmaking body may be expected to produce based on sociodemographic trends in public opinion. Although 47% of participants in the Pew study approved of PAD, for example, it is illegal in 41 states. This disparity may have to do with other ways in which the sociodemographic characteristics of lawmakers differ from those of the general public. For example, only one person out of the 534 in the 116th Congress identified as having no religious affiliation, although 23% of Americans say they do not belong to any faith tradition (Pew Research Center, 2019).

In the final step of my analysis, I tested two possible explanations for the racial and ethnic differences in attitudes about euthanasia. First, the survey asked a question about respondents' trust in health care professionals. On average, persons of color say that they trust their health care professionals as much as non-Hispanic Whites do, but they are not as likely to trust that their health care professionals will engage in specific appropriate practices such as refraining from unnecessary tests and making referrals to specialists, and persons of color report fewer positive interactions with their health care providers than non-Hispanic Whites do (Halbert et al., 2006; Stepanikova et al., 2006). Historically, and even recently, persons of color have been subjected to illicit medical experimentation (Washington, 2006), systemic racism in healthcare (Feagin & Bennefield, 2014), and the use of medicine as a means of social control (Roberts, 1999).

The Pew survey question read

> How much attention do you think doctors and nurses pay to instructions from patients about whether or not they want treatment to keep

them alive? Do you think doctors and nurses pay a lot of attention, some attention, or very little attention to patients' instructions?

Overall, 39% said that doctors and nurses pay a lot of attention, 45% said that they pay some attention, and 14% said that they pay very little attention. There were significant differences, however, in the opinions of White non-Hispanic, Black non-Hispanic, and Hispanic survey participants. Twelve percent of White non-Hispanic people were concerned that doctors and nurses pay very little attention to patient preferences, whereas 29% of Hispanic participants voiced this concern. Among White non-Hispanic people, 42% believed that doctors and nurses pay a lot of attention, while only 34% of Black non-Hispanic people had this high degree of confidence in their health care providers.

Second, the survey asked questions about the participant's recent experience with end-of-life situations. Non-Hispanic Blacks, in particular, experience more deaths across the life course than do non-Hispanic Whites (Umberson, 2017; Umberson et al., 2017). Experiences with death, especially with the decedent's physical pain and use of life-sustaining treatments, shape individuals' attitudes and beliefs about end-of-life care (Carr, 2012).

Participants reported whether "you had any personal experience in the last five years with a relative or close friend suffering from a terminal illness or in a coma?" Participants who said yes went on to answer "Did the issue of withholding life-sustaining treatment come up, or not?" I used this information to generate three categories of people: those with no recent experience with a very ill person, those with experience with a very ill person but no issues concerning withholding life-sustaining treatment, and those with experience with a very ill person where withholding life-sustaining treatment came up. In the subsample of people with the four most common attitudes towards euthanasia, 53% had no experience with a very ill loved on in the past five years. Among the 47% who did, withholding life-sustaining treatment did not come up for 42%, and it did come up for 58%.

There were racial/ethnic differences in this experience, although they were not consistent with other national data, perhaps due to the younger age of persons of color in the Pew survey. Among White non-Hispanic participants, 50% had no experience in the past five years, while knowing a very ill person was significantly less common among persons of color. Fifty-six percent of Black non-Hispanic participants and 61% of Hispanic participants had not experienced the serious illness of a relative or close friend. Among people who had this experience, there were no significant racial/ethnic differences in whether the experience had included decision-making about life-sustaining treatment.

Finally, I added the measures of trust in health care professionals and experience with death to the regression model presented above. Table 8.7 shows the results of this analysis for race/ethnicity, trust in health care professionals, experience with death, and quality of life beliefs. Gender, educational attainment, region, income, country of birth, religious affiliation, and age were also included in the model, but

TABLE 8.7 Multiple Multinomial Logistic Regression of Racial/Ethnic Differences in Attitudes toward Euthanasia Given Trust in Health Care Providers and Experience with Death, Results Presented as Predicted Probabilities, 2013 Pew Research Center Survey on Aging and Longevity, $N = 1,056$

	Oppose passive and active euthanasia	*Approve passive, oppose active*	*Approve passive and suicide, oppose PAD*	*Approve passive and active euthanasia*
Race/ethnicity				
White non-Hispanic	6	15	15	64
Black non-Hispanic	32	9	20	39
Hispanic	15	8	26	51
Potential mediators				
A lot of trust in health care providers	14	17	16	54
Very little to no trust in health care providers	14	14	15	58
No recent experience with death	11	13	18	58
Experience, without life-sustaining decision	8	12	20	60
Experience, with life-sustaining decision	7	13	15	65

the results for these variables are not shown in Table 8.7. Table 8.A3, in the Appendix, shows the complete results of the regression analysis in the form of odds ratios.

The analysis shows that neither trust in health care providers nor experience with death explained the racial and ethnic differences in attitudes about euthanasia. The differences among White non-Hispanic, Black non-Hispanic, and Hispanic participants persisted after accounting for these factors. These results are surprising, but consistent with those of a growing body of empirical studies, in which racial and ethnic differences in end-of-life values and choices persisted net of the importance respondents placed on life extension (Huang et al., 2016), religious belief (Koss, 2018), experiences of racial or ethnic discrimination, and trust in medical providers (Koss & Baker, 2017).

Limitations

No single study that fails to find a statistical connection between variables can provide sufficient evidence to conclude that these factors do not account for racial and ethnic differences, because limitations in the data and analysis may account for the results. First, this analysis has low statistical power in places; for example, only 7% of Hispanics, or 42 participants, approved of both passive and active euthanasia. This small sample may not be representative of Hispanics who approve of euthanasia in the total adult population. Second, the way a survey question is worded influences how people answer that question. The Pew Center questions use the word suicide, a strongly negative word, when referring to PAD. The newer term medical aid-in-dying may be less well known, but may also be less stigmatizing. Third, closed-ended, forced-choice survey questions may be insufficient to assess individuals' complex and nuanced views about these issues. A more qualitative design that permitted participants to explain their experiences and their opinions may have yielded richer answers.

Future Directions

However frustrating, these null findings are a step towards identifying the sources of racial and ethnic variation in public opinion, which is important because race is so often a marker of discriminatory treatment in the U.S. That is, implicit in both fundamental cause theory and public conversation is the assumption that if persons of color had more favorable experiences with death and the health care system, then they would approve of euthanasia at the same rates that White people do. This assumption is based in a deficits model of thinking: People of color have poorer interactions with the health care system than Whites, and more experiences of death, and so these vulnerabilities must necessarily have negative effects on their attitudes. But perhaps racial and ethnic differences in attitudes towards euthanasia are not due to discrimination in the ways that scholars have hypothesized. For example, perhaps more frequent experience of death increases the value of life among people of color (King et al., 2009). Future research should pivot towards assessing the strengths of communities of color. Perhaps racial and ethnic differences in attitudes towards euthanasia are due to positive influences that people of color experience more often than White Americans do.

Summary

The legal status of active euthanasia, and even passive euthanasia in specific cases, is controversial in the U.S. Public opinion and law are increasingly accepting forms of voluntary active euthanasia, particularly physician-assisted death (also called medical aid in dying). However, active euthanasia is illegal in most of the U.S., and public opinion includes significant minorities of people who are staunchly opposed, especially among communities of color. Analysis of the Survey of Aging and Longevity shows that in 2013, all forms of euthanasia were more acceptable to White non-Hispanic Americans than to Black non-Hispanic and Hispanic Americans. These three groups also expressed different levels of trust in health care providers and different experiences with death. However, racial and ethnic differences in opinion about euthanasia persisted even after accounting for these varied sociocultural factors.

Data Appendix

As part of the Religion and Public Life Project, the Pew Research Center sought to draw conclusions about U.S. persons aged 18 years and older in the year 2013. In order to do so, they drew a random sample from this population. Potential participants were contacted at random from lists of landline and cellular telephone

TABLE 8.A1 Characteristics of Participants by Racial/Ethnic Subgroup, 2013 Pew Research Center Survey on Aging and Longevity, $N = 1{,}832$

	White non-Hispanic[A]	*Black non-Hispanic*[B]	*Hispanic*[C]	*Significant subgroup differences*
Female	53%	55%	52%	none
Educational attainment				
Less than high school	4%	11%	23%	AB, AC, BC
High school graduate	23%	25%	31%	AB, AC
Some college	28%	30%	22%	none
BA or more	46%	25%	23%	AB, AC
Region				
Northeast	13%	19%	16%	AB
Midwest	20%	15%	9%	AC
South	45%	56%	40%	AB, BC
West	22%	10%	36%	AB, AC, BC
Median income	\$50,000–74,999	\$30,000–39,999	\$30,000–39,999	AB, AC
Foreign-born	4%	7%	49%	AC, BC
Religious affiliation				
Mainline Protestant	23%	19%	7%	AC, BC
Evangelical Protestant	30%	54%	15%	AB, AC, BC
Roman Catholic	20%	6%	51%	AB, AC, BC
Other affiliation	9%	5%	3%	AC
Unaffiliated	19%	17%	23%	none
Average age in years	54.7(SD = 17.9)	48.3(SD = 17.7)	42.5(SD = 16.4)	AB, AC, BC

Notes
Analysis of variance (ANOVA) tests were used to assess subgroup differences. Significant differences ($p < 0.05$) are denoted as AB: White non-Hispanic vs. Black non-Hispanic; AC: White non-Hispanic vs. Hispanic; and BC: Black non-Hispanic vs. Hispanic.

TABLE 8.A2 Multiple Multinomial Logistic Regression of Racial/Ethnic Differences in Attitudes toward Euthanasia, Results Presented as Odds Ratios with 95% Confidence Intervals, 2013 Pew Research Center Survey on Aging and Longevity, $N = 1{,}056$

	Oppose active and passive euthanasia	*Approve passive, oppose active*	*Approve passive and suicide, oppose physician-assistance*
	Approve active and passive euthanasia		
	Odds Ratio (CI)	*Odds Ratio (CI)*	*Odds Ratio (CI)*
Race/ethnicity (reference: White non-Hispanic)			
Black non-Hispanic	7.27*** (3.99–13.26)	0.92 (0.46–1.81)	2.34** (1.27–4.31)
Hispanic	3.37*** (1.67–6.79)	0.66 (0.27–1.62)	2.24** (1.20–4.15)
Female	1.03 (0.64–1.67)	1.34 (0.88–2.06)	0.92 (0.61–1.39)
Educational attainment (reference: BA or more)			
Less than high school	8.13*** (2.45–26.96)	1.22 (0.24–6.06)	7.30*** (2.33–22.81)
High school graduate	3.02*** (1.61–5.67)	1.76* (1.01–3.10)	2.18** (1.27–3.74)
Some college	1.58 (0.85–2.94)	1.11 (0.66–1.87)	1.06 (0.62–1.81)
Region (reference: Northeast)			
Midwest	1.22 (0.52–2.85)	2.15* (1.02–4.52)	2.91** (1.39–6.08)
South	1.59 (0.80–3.18)	1.74 (0.89–3.43)	1.92 (0.97–3.80)
West	1.15 (0.52–2.54)	0.88 (0.39–1.97)	1.82 (0.86–3.85)
Income (1 = less than \$10,000; 9 = \$150,000 or more)	0.86** (0.77–0.96)	0.92 (0.84–1.02)	0.91 (0.83–1.01)
Foreign-born	3.23*** (1.57–6.64)	1.10 (0.41–2.90)	1.27 (0.59–2.72)
Religious affiliation (reference: Mainline Protestant)			
Evangelical Protestant	3.89*** (1.97–7.69)	6.85*** (3.83–12.24)	2.16** (1.22–3.82)
Roman Catholic	1.38 (0.63–3.04)	1.25 (0.64–2.46)	1.07 (0.58–1.97)
Other affiliation	2.44 (0.91–6.51)	2.10 (0.88–5.01)	0.69 (0.24–1.96)
Unaffiliated	0.38* (0.16–0.88)	0.31** (0.13–0.77)	0.45* (0.24–0.86)
Age (years)	0.99 (0.98–1.00)	1.01 (0.99–1.02)	1.00 (0.99–1.01)

Note
Statistical significance denoted as $^{***}p < 0.001$; $^{**}p < 0.01$; $^{*}p < 0.05$.

TABLE 8.A3 Multiple Multinomial Logistic Regression of Racial/Ethnic Differences in Attitudes toward Euthanasia Given Trust in Health Care Providers and Experience with Death, Results Presented as Odds Ratios with 95% Confidence Intervals 2013 Pew Research Center Survey on Aging and Longevity, $N = 1{,}056$

	Oppose active and passive euthanasia	*Approve passive, oppose active*	*Approve passive and suicide, oppose physician-assistance*
	Approve active and passive euthanasia		
	Odds Ratio (CI)	*Odds Ratio (CI)*	*Odds Ratio (CI)*
Race/ethnicity (reference: White non-Hispanic)			
Black non-Hispanic	8.51*** (4.54–15.93)	0.97 (0.48–1.93)	2.19* (1.16–4.12)
Hispanic	3.06** (1.49–6.31)	0.67 (0.27–1.67)	2.19* (1.17–4.09)
Potential mediators			
Trust in health care providers (1 = a lot; 3 = very little to none)	0.95 (0.68–1.34)	0.81 (0.59–1.12)	0.92 (0.68–1.24)
Recent experience with death (reference: none)			
Yes, without life-sustaining decision	0.71 (0.38–1.35)	0.87 (0.49–1.54)	1.08 (0.64–1.83)
Yes, with life-sustaining decision	0.58 (0.32–1.05)	0.89 (0.55–1.44)	0.74 (0.45–1.21)
Functional quality of life (0 = least important; 4 = most important)	0.79** (0.67–0.92)	0.94 (0.81–1.08)	0.92 (0.80–1.06)
Female	1.10 (0.68–1.81)	1.38 (0.89–2.14)	0.98 (0.65–1.49)
Educational attainment (reference: BA or more)			
Less than high school	7.44*** (2.17–25.57)	1.55 (0.31–7.85)	6.45** (2.02–20.67)
High school graduate	3.02*** (1.61–5.67)	1.80 (1.00–3.23)	2.14** (1.23–3.72)
Some college	1.60 (0.85–3.01)	1.15 (0.68–1.95)	1.07 (0.63–1.83)
Region (reference: Northeast)			
Midwest	1.56 (0.65–3.74)	2.18* (1.03–4.64)	3.04** (1.44–6.39)
South	1.84 (0.90–3.76)	1.69 (0.85–3.36)	1.92 (0.96–3.83)
West	1.30 (0.57–2.96)	0.94 (0.42–2.12)	1.86 (0.88–3.96)

Income (1 = less than $10,000; 9 = $150,000 or more)	0.84** (0.75–0.95)	0.91 (0.82–1.01)	0.91 (0.82–1.00)
Foreign-born	3.12** (1.49–6.54)	1.16 (0.43–3.10)	1.32 (0.61–2.83)
Religious affiliation (reference: Mainline Protestant)			
Evangelical Protestant	4.01*** (1.99–8.08)	6.65*** (3.71–11.94)	2.36** (1.32–4.21)
Roman Catholic	1.59 (0.71–3.56)	1.21 (0.61–2.41)	1.13 (0.60–2.10)
Other affiliation	2.44 (0.89–6.73)	2.06 (0.86–4.93)	0.71 (0.25–2.05)
Unaffiliated	0.42 (0.18–1.00)	0.22** (0.08–0.61)	0.50* (0.26–0.96)
Age (years)	0.98 (0.96–1.00)	1.01 (0.99–1.02)	1.00 (0.98–1.01)

Note
Statistical significance denoted as ***$p < 0.001$; **$p < 0.01$; *$p < 0.05$.

numbers. The sample thus excludes anyone who did not have a telephone, while people who had more than one telephone number had a higher probability of being contacted. Pew selected a larger proportion of telephone numbers from counties with larger proportions of non-Hispanic Black and Hispanic residents, so as to increase the representation of these groups in the study. The Pew Center did not release the number of potential participants they contacted in order to generate their sample. Along with the released data, the Pew Center released a weighting variable that can be used to adjust estimates for design effects, including probability of having a telephone, county in which the phone number is registered, and non-response. I did not use that weighting variable in the analyses presented here.

Overall, 4,006 participants responded to the survey. However, most survey modules, including the questions about euthanasia, were asked of a random half of the sample. The sample size for the analyses in this chapter is 1,832, after eliminating participants who were not asked the relevant questions and participants who identified as a race or ethnicity other than non-Hispanic White, non-Hispanic Black, or Hispanic. The margin of error is approximately 2.9%, which means that the sample represents the U.S. population quite well. For example, 69% of participants said that there are circumstances where a patient should be allowed to die. Had the Pew Center been able to ask everyone in the U.S. aged 18 or older, between 66.1% and 71.9% would have agreed with this statement. Readers should be aware that the margins of error are higher for racial/ethnic subgroups because margin of error is derived from total group size. For non-Hispanic Blacks, the margin of error is 7.0%; for Hispanics, it is 6.7%; and for non-Hispanic Whites, it is 3.8%.

Note

1. Currently, the term *medical aid in dying* is popular because advocates object to the use of the stigmatized word *suicide*. However, I use the term PAD because *physician-assisted* is more precise than *medical aid* with regard to the actors and actions occurring.

References

Albaladejo, A. (2019). Fear of assisted dying: Could it lead to euthanasia on demand or worsen access to palliative care? *British Medical Journal, 364*, 1852. https://doi.org/10.1136/bmj.l852.

American Medical Association. (2019). *Code of medical ethic opinion 5.8*. www.ama-assn.org/delivering-care/ethics/euthanasia.

Attell, B. (2015). *Social change in attitudes toward euthanasia and suicide for terminally ill persons, 1977–2014: An age-period-cohort analysis* [Master's thesis, Georgia State University]. https://scholarworks.gsu.edu/sociology_theses/55.

Barry, R. (2017). *Breaking the thread of life: On rational suicide*. Routledge. https://doi.org/10.4324/9781315082004.

Bélanger, E., Towers, A., Wright, D. K., Chen, Y., Tradounsky, G., & Macdonald, M. E. (2019). Of dilemmas and tensions: A qualitative study of palliative care physicians' positions regarding voluntary active euthanasia in Quebec, Canada. *Journal of Medical Ethics*, *45*(1), 48–53. https://doi.org/10.1136/medethics-2017-104339.

Blanke, C., LeBlanc, M., Hershman, D., Ellis, L., & Meyskens, F. (2017). Characterizing 18 years of the Death with Dignity Act in Oregon. *Journal of the American Medical Association Oncology*, *3*(10), 1403–1406. https://doi.org/10.1001/jamaoncol.2017.0243.

Bor, J. (2017). Diverging life expectancies and voting patterns in the 2016 US presidential election. *American Journal of Public Health*, *107*(10), 1560–1562. https://doi.org/10.2105/AJPH.2017.303945.

Boudreau, J. D. (2011). Physician-assisted suicide and euthanasia: Can you even imagine teaching medical students how to end their patients' lives? *The Permanente Journal*, *15*(4), 79–84. https://doi.org/10.7812/tpp/11-099

Buchbinder, M. (2018a). Choreographing death: A social phenomenology of medical aid-in-dying in the United States. *Medical Anthropology Quarterly*, *32*(4), 481–497. https://doi.org/10.1111/maq.12468.

Buchbinder, M. (2018b). Access to aid-in-dying in the United States: Shifting the debate from rights to justice. *American Journal of Public Health*, *108*(6), 754–759. https://doi.org/10.2105/AJPH.2018.304352.

Buchbinder, M. (2019). The power of suggestion: Disclosure ideologies and medically assisted death. *Medicine Anthropology Theory*, *6*(1), 5–29. https://doi.org/10.17157/mat.6.1.645.

Buchbinder, M., Ojo, E., Knio, L., & Brassfield, E. R. (2018). Caregivers' experiences with medical aid-in-dying in Vermont: A qualitative study. *Journal of Pain and Symptom Management*, *56*(6), 936–943. https://doi.org/10.1016/j.jpainsymman.2018.08.010.

Burgat, C., & Hunt, C. (2018). *Congress in 2019*. Brookings Institution. www.brookings.edu/blog/fixgov/2018/12/28/congress-in-2019-the-2nd-most-educated-and-least-politically-experienced-house-freshman-class/.

Cain, C. L., & McCleskey, S. (2019). Expanded definitions of the 'good death'? Race, ethnicity and medical aid in dying. *Sociology of Health & Illness*, *41*(6), 1175–1191. https://doi.org/10.1111/1467-9566.12903.

Caplan, A. L., Blank, R. H., & Merrick, J. C. (2012). *Compelled compassion: Government intervention in the treatment of critically ill newborns*. Springer Science & Business Media.

Carr, D. (2012). "I don't want to die like that ...": The impact of significant others' death quality on advance care planning. *The Gerontologist*, *52*(6), 770–781. https://doi.org/10.1093/geront/gns051.

Chambaere, K., & Bernheim, J. L. (2015). Does legal physician-assisted dying impede development of palliative care? The Belgian and Benelux experience. *Journal of Medical Ethics*, *41*(8), 657–660. https://doi.org/10.1136/medethics-2014-102116.

Charatan, F. (1999). Dr Kevorkian found guilty of second degree murder. *British Medical Journal*, *318*(7189), 962.

Cherlin, A. J. (2018). Psychological health and socioeconomic status among non-Hispanic whites. *Proceedings of the National Academy of Sciences of the United States of America*, *115*(28), 7176–7178. https://doi.org/10.1073/pnas.1808753115.

Chervenak, F. A., Mccullough, L. B., & Arabin, B. (2006). Why the Groningen Protocol should be rejected. *Hastings Center Report*, *36*(5), 30–33. https://doi.org/10.1353/hcr.2006.0073.

Clark, A. E. (2005). The right to die: The broken road from Quinlan to Schiavo. *Loyola University Chicago Law Journal*, *37*, 385.

Cooper, S. (2010). Taking no for an answer: Refusal of life-sustaining treatment. *American Medical Association Journal of Ethics*, *12*(6), 444–449. https://doi.org/10.1001/virtualmentor.2010.12.6.ccas2-1006.

Dan, B., Fonteyne, C., & Cléty, S. C. de. (2014). Self-requested euthanasia for children in Belgium. *The Lancet, 383*(9918), 671–672. https://doi.org/10.1016/S0140-6736(14)60110-0.

Davis, D. S. (2014). Alzheimer disease and pre-emptive suicide. *Journal of Medical Ethics, 40*(8), 543–549. https://doi.org/10.1136/medethics-2012-101022.

Dierickx, S., Deliens, L., Cohen, J., & Chambaere, K. (2018). Involvement of palliative care in euthanasia practice in a context of legalized euthanasia: A population-based mortality follow-back study. *Palliative Medicine, 32*(1), 114–122. https://doi.org/10.1177/0269216317727158.

Dixon, N. (1998). On the difference between physician-assisted suicide and active euthanasia. *The Hastings Center Report, 28*(5), 25–29.

Duncan, O. D., & Parmelee, L. F. (2006). Trends in public approval of euthanasia and suicide in the US, 1947–2003. *Journal of Medical Ethics, 32*(5), 266–272. https://doi.org/10.1136/jme.2004.011072.

Dwyer, D. (2019, December 20). Across New England are families who have lost loved ones to opioids. These 4 parents lost more than one child. *Boston Globe*. www.boston.com/news/local-news/2019/12/20/parents-multiple-children-fatal-overdoses-opioid-crisis-new-england.

Feagin, J., & Bennefield, Z. (2014). Systemic racism and U.S. health care. *Social Science & Medicine, 103*, 7–14. https://doi.org/10.1016/j.socscimed.2013.09.006.

Gostin, L. O., & Roberts, A. E. (2016). Physician-assisted dying: A turning point? *Journal of the American Medical Association, 315*(3), 249–250. https://doi.org/10.1001/jama.2015.16586.

Grodin, M. A., Miller, E. L., & Kelly, J. I. (2017). The Nazi physicians as leaders in eugenics and "euthanasia:" Lessons for today. *American Journal of Public Health, 108*(1), 53–57. https://doi.org/10.2105/AJPH.2017.304120.

Gurschick, L., Mayer, D. K., & Hanson, L. C. (2015). Palliative sedation: An analysis of international guidelines and position statements. *American Journal of Hospice and Palliative Medicine®, 32*(6), 660–671. https://doi.org/10.1177/1049909114533002.

Halbert, C. H., Armstrong, K., Gandy, O. H., & Shaker, L. (2006). Racial differences in trust in health care providers. *Archives of Internal Medicine, 166*(8), 896–901. https://doi.org/10.1001/archinte.166.8.896.

Hedberg, K., & New, C. (2017). Oregon's Death With Dignity Act: 20 years of experience to inform the debate. *Annals of Internal Medicine, 167*(8), 579. https://doi.org/10.7326/M17-2300.

Hedegaard, H., Curtin, S. C., & Warner, M. (2018). *Suicide mortality in the United States, 1999–2017* (NCHS Data Brief No. 330). National Center for Health Statistics. www.cdc.gov/nchs/products/databriefs/db330.htm.

Huang, I. A., Neuhaus, J. M., & Chiong, W. (2016). Racial and ethnic differences in advance directive possession: Role of demographic factors, religious affiliation, and personal health values in a national survey of older adults. *Journal of Palliative Medicine, 19*(2), 149–156. https://doi.org/10.1089/jpm.2015.0326.

Iait, M. (2020, January 3). Judge rules that doctors can take baby off life support against mother's wishes. *Washington Post*. www.washingtonpost.com/health/2020/01/03/after-hospital-mother-disagree-court-had-rule-who-decides-when-child-dies/.

Joseph, J. (2005). The 1942 'euthanasia' debate in the American Journal of Psychiatry. *History of Psychiatry, 16*(2), 171–179. https://doi.org/10.1177/0957154X05047004.

Jotkowitz, A. B., & Glick, S. (2006). The Groningen protocol: Another perspective. *Journal of Medical Ethics, 32*(3), 157–158. https://doi.org/10.1136/jme.2005.012476.

Jotkowitz, A., Glick, S., & Gesundheit, B. (2008). A case against justified non-voluntary active euthanasia (The Groningen Protocol). *The American Journal of Bioethics*, *8*(11), 23–26. https://doi.org/10.1080/15265160802513085.

Keown, J. (2018). *Euthanasia, ethics and public policy: An argument against legalisation*. Cambridge University Press.

King, L. A., Hicks, J. A., & Abdelkhalik, J. (2009). Death, life, scarcity, and value: An alternative perspective on the meaning of death. *Psychological Science*, *20*(12), 1459–1462. https://doi.org/10.1111/j.1467-9280.2009.02466.x.

Kopelman, L. M. (2005). Are the 21-year-old Baby Doe rules misunderstood or mistaken? *Pediatrics*, *115*(3), 797–802. https://doi.org/10.1542/peds.2004-2326.

Koss, C. S. (2018). Does religiosity account for lower rates of advance care planning by older African Americans? *The Journals of Gerontology: Series B*, *73*(4), 687–695. https://doi.org/10.1093/geronb/gbw155.

Koss, C. S., & Baker, T. A. (2017). A question of trust: Does mistrust or perceived discrimination account for race disparities in advance directive completion? *Innovation in Aging*, *1*(1). https://doi.org/10.1093/geroni/igx017.

Lam, M., Lam, H. R., Agarwal, A., Chow, R., Chow, S., Chow, E., De Longhi, C., Wan, A., & Henry, B. (2017). Clinicians' views on palliative sedation for existential suffering: A systematic review and thematic synthesis of qualitative studies. *Journal of Pain Management*, *10*(1), 31–40.

LoPresti, M. A., Dement, F., & Gold, H. T. (2016). End-of-life care for people with cancer from ethnic minority groups: A systematic review. *American Journal of Hospice and Palliative Medicine*, *33*(3), 291–305. https://doi.org/10.1177/1049909114565658.

Maeda, I., Morita, T., Yamaguchi, T., Inoue, S., Ikenaga, M., Matsumoto, Y., Sekine, R., Yamaguchi, T., Hirohashi, T., Tajima, T., Tatara, R., Watanabe, H., Otani, H., Takigawa, C., Matsuda, Y., Nagaoka, H., Mori, M., Tei, Y., Kikuchi, A., … Kinoshita, H. (2016). Effect of continuous deep sedation on survival in patients with advanced cancer (J-Proval): A propensity score-weighted analysis of a prospective cohort study. *The Lancet Oncology*, *17*(1), 115–122. https://doi.org/10.1016/S1470-2045(15)00401-5.

Maltoni, M., Scarpi, E., Rosati, M., Derni, S., Fabbri, L., Martini, F., Amadori, D., & Nanni, O. (2012). Palliative sedation in end-of-life care and survival: A systematic review. *Journal of Clinical Oncology*, *30*(12), 1378-1383. https://doi.org/10.1200/JCO.2011.37.3795.

Monnat, S. M., Peters, D. J., Berg, M. T., & Hochstetler, A. (2019). Using Census data to understand county-level differences in overall drug mortality and opioid-related mortality by opioid type. *American Journal of Public Health*, *109*(8), 1084–1091. https://doi.org/10.2105/AJPH.2019.305136.

Morita, T., Tsuneto, S., & Shima, Y. (2002). Definition of sedation for symptom relief: A systematic literature review and a proposal of operational criteria. *Journal of Pain and Symptom Management*, *24*(4), 447–453. https://doi.org/10.1016/S0885-3924(02)00499-2.

Nair-Collins, M. (2017). Medical futility and involuntary passive euthanasia. *Perspectives in Biology and Medicine*, *60*(3), 415–422. https://doi.org/10.1353/pbm.2018.0017.

National Institute of Mental Health. (2019). *Suicide*. www.nimh.nih.gov/health/statistics/suicide.shtml#part_155137.

Ollove, M. (2018, July 30). Assisted suicide is controversial, but palliative sedation is legal and offers peace. *Washington Post*. www.washingtonpost.com/national/health-science/assisted-suicide-is-controversial-but-palliative-sedation-is-legal-and-offers-peace/2018/07/27/e9b02cf8-8922-11e8-8aea-86e88ae760d8_story.html.

Oregon Health Authority. (2020). *Death with Dignity reporting forms and instructions*. www.oregon.gov/oha/PH/PROVIDERPARTNERRESOURCES/EVALUATIONRESEARCH/DEATHWITHDIGNITYACT/Pages/pasforms.aspx.

Papavasiliou, E. (Evie), & Payne, S. (2015). Unaddressed biases in reported prevalence of continuous deep sedation until death. *Journal of Clinical Epidemiology, 68*(10), 1241–1242. https://doi.org/10.1016/j.jclinepi.2014.11.007.

Periyakoil, V.S., Kraemer, H., & Neri, E. (2016). Multi-ethnic attitudes toward physician-assisted death in California and Hawaii. *Journal of Palliative Medicine, 19*(10), 1060–1065. https://doi.org/10.1089/jpm.2016.0160.

Peters, D. J., Monnat, S. M., Hochstetler, A. L., & Berg, M. T. (2019). The opioid hydra: Understanding overdose mortality epidemics and syndemics across the rural-urban continuum. *Rural Sociology*. https://doi.org/10.1111/ruso.12307.

Petrillo, L.A., Dzeng, E., Harrison, K. L., Forbes, L., Scribner, B., & Koenig, B.A. (2017). How California prepared for implementation of physician-assisted death: A primer. *American Journal of Public Health, 107*(6), 883–888. https://doi.org/10.2105/AJPH.2017.303755.

Pew Research Center. (2013a). *Religious groups' views on end-of-life issues*. www.pewforum.org/2013/11/21/religious-groups-views-on-end-of-life-issues/.

Pew Research Center. (2013b). *To end our days*. www.pewforum.org/2013/11/21/to-end-our-days/.

Pew Research Center. (2013c). *Views on end-of-life medical treatments*. www.pewforum.org/2013/11/21/views-on-end-of-life-medical-treatments/.

Pew Research Center. (2019). *Religious affiliation of the 116th Congress*. www.pewforum.org/2019/01/03/faith-on-the-hill-116/.

Pope, T. M. (2008). Involuntary passive euthanasia in U.S. courts: Reassessing the judicial treatment of medical futility cases. *Marquette Elder's Advisor, 9*(2).

Putman, M. S., Yoon, J. D., Rasinski, K. A., & Curlin, F. A. (2013). Intentional sedation to unconsciousness at the end of life: Findings from a national physician survey. *Journal of Pain and Symptom Management, 46*(3), 326–334. https://doi.org/10.1016/j.jpainsymman.2012.09.007.

Quill, T. E. (2005). Terri Schiavo – A tragedy compounded. *New England Journal of Medicine, 352*(16), 1630–1633. https://doi.org/10.1056/NEJMp058062.

Roberts, D. E. (1999). *Killing the Black body: Race, reproduction, and the meaning of liberty*. Vintage.

Rodrigues, P., Crokaert, J., & Gastmans, C. (2018). Palliative sedation for existential suffering: A systematic review of argument-based ethics literature. *Journal of Pain and Symptom Management, 55*(6), 1577–1590. https://doi.org/10.1016/j.jpainsymman.2018.01.013.

Schildmann, E., & Schildmann, J. (2014). Palliative sedation therapy: A systematic literature review and critical appraisal of available guidance on indication and decision making. *Journal of Palliative Medicine, 17*(5), 601–611. https://doi.org/10.1089/jpm.2013.0511.

Schur, S., Weixler, D., Gabl, C., Kreye, G., Likar, R., Masel, E. K., Mayrhofer, M., Reiner, F., Schmidmayr, B., Kirchheiner, K., & Watzke, H. H. (2016). Sedation at the end of life: A nation-wide study in palliative care units in Austria. *BMC Palliative Care, 15*(1), 50. https://doi.org/10.1186/s12904-016-0121-8.

Siegel, A. M., Sisti, D. A., & Caplan, A. L. (2014). Pediatric euthanasia in Belgium: Disturbing developments. *Journal of the American Medical Association, 311*(19), 1963–1964. https://doi.org/10.1001/jama.2014.4257.

Stein, E. M., Gennuso, K. P., Ugboaja, D. C., & Remington, P. L. (2017). The epidemic of despair among white Americans: Trends in the leading causes of premature death, 1999–2015. *American Journal of Public Health, 107*(10), 1541–1547. https://doi.org/10.2105/AJPH.2017.303941.

Stepanikova, I., Mollborn, S., Cook, K. S., Thom, D. H., & Kramer, R. M. (2006). Patients' race, ethnicity, language, and trust in a physician. *Journal of Health and Social Behavior, 47*(4), 390–405. https://doi.org/10.1177/002214650604700406.

Sulmasy, D. P., Ely, E. W., & Sprung, C. L. (2016). Euthanasia and physician-assisted suicide. *Journal of the American Medical Association, 316*(15), 1600–1600. https://doi.org/10.1001/jama.2016.14077.

Sulmasy, D. P., Travaline, J. M., Mitchell, L. A., & Ely, E. W. (2016). Non-faith-based arguments against physician-assisted suicide and euthanasia. *The Linacre Quarterly, 83*(3), 246–257. https://doi.org/10.1080/00243639.2016.1201375.

Terry, P. B. (1995). Euthanasia and assisted suicide. *Mayo Clinic Proceedings, 70*(2), 189–192. https://doi.org/10.4065/70.2.189.

Tschirhart, E. C., Du, Q., & Kelley, A. S. (2014). Factors influencing the use of intensive procedures at the end of life. *Journal of the American Geriatrics Society, 62*(11), 2088–2094. https://doi.org/10.1111/jgs.13104.

Umberson, D. (2017). Black deaths matter: Race, relationship loss, and effects on survivors. *Journal of Health and Social Behavior, 58*(4), 405–420. https://doi.org/10.1177/0022146517739317.

Umberson, D., Olson, J. S., Crosnoe, R., Liu, H., Pudrovska, T., & Donnelly, R. (2017). Death of family members as an overlooked source of racial disadvantage in the United States. *Proceedings of the National Academy of Sciences, 114*(5), 915–920. https://doi.org/10.1073/pnas.1605599114.

United States Senate. (2019). *Ethnic diversity in the Senate.* www.senate.gov/senators/EthnicDiversityintheSenate.htm.

Ventafridda, V., Ripamonti, C., De Conno, F., Tamburini, M., & Cassileth, B. R. (1990). Symptom prevalence and control during cancer patients' last days of life. *Journal of Palliative Care, 6*(3), 7–11. https://doi.org/10.1177/082585979000600303.

Verhagen, A. A. (2014). Neonatal euthanasia: Lessons from the Groningen Protocol. *Seminars in Fetal and Neonatal Medicine, 19*(5), 296–299. https://doi.org/10.1016/j.siny.2014.08.002.

Verhagen, A. A., & Sauer, P. J. J. (2005a). The Groningen Protocol – Euthanasia in severely ill newborns. *New England Journal of Medicine, 352*(10), 959–962. https://doi.org/10.1056/NEJMp058026.

Verhagen, A. A., & Sauer, P. J. J. (2005b). End-of-life decisions in newborns: An approach from the Netherlands. *Pediatrics, 116*(3), 736–739. https://doi.org/10.1542/peds.2005-0014.

Washington, H. A. (2006). *Medical apartheid: The dark history of medical experimentation on Black Americans from colonial times to the present.* Doubleday.

Washington State Department of Health. (2019). *Death with Dignity data.* www.doh.wa.gov/YouandYourFamily/IllnessandDisease/DeathwithDignityAct/DeathwithDignityData.

Werth Jr., J. L. (1996). *Rational suicide? Implications for mental health professionals.* Taylor & Francis.

Winter, L., & Parks, S. M. (2012). Acceptors and rejecters of life-sustaining treatment: Differences in advance care planning characteristics. *Journal of Applied Gerontology, 31*(6), 734–742. https://doi.org/10.1177/0733464811399079.

Zalsman, G., Hawton, K., Wasserman, D., van Heeringen, K., Arensman, E., Sarchiapone, M., Carli, V., Höschl, C., Barzilay, R., Balazs, J., Purebl, G., Kahn, J. P., Sáiz, P. A., Lipsicas, C. B., Bobes, J., Cozman, D., Hegerl, U., & Zohar, J. (2016). Suicide prevention strategies revisited: 10-year systematic review. *The Lancet Psychiatry, 3*(7), 646–659. https://doi.org/10.1016/S2215-0366(16)30030-X.

Zraick, K. (2020, January 2). Texas judge rules that hospital can take baby off life support. *The New York Times.* www.nytimes.com/2020/01/02/us/texas-infant-life-support.html.

CONCLUSIONS

This book has focused on predictable death, or death after the age of 65 from one or more chronic illnesses. Three-quarters of deaths in the U.S. each year meet this description (S. L. Murphy et al., 2018). Predictable death makes the entire life course more foreseeable. Beginning in adolescence, most people can hazard a reasonable estimate of their longevity (Mirowsky, 1997; Swisher & Warner, 2013). Young people can assume the responsibilities of adulthood more slowly than in the past, and they can devote time to higher education and to finding a compatible life partner (Arnett, 2000). In midlife, people can tend their health: People who expect to live to old age exercise more regularly than people who expect to die, and also adhere better to physical therapy regimens aimed at rehabilitation from a disease, injury, or surgery (Kahana et al., 2005; Levy et al., 2012). Adults in midlife can save money for retirement and for the long-term care that is a consequence of chronic illness.

The end of life has become a stage in the life course, like infancy or adolescence (Carr & Luth, 2019). Older adults have valid perceptions of how close they are to death (Kotter-Grühn et al., 2010). People generally do not want to live forever, but rather only so long as their health is good, their friends and family are also living, they can learn new things and meet new people, and they can make a difference in the world (Cicirelli, 2011; Ekerdt et al., 2017). Then people can plan for death, arranging what kinds of care they would like, what they would like to accomplish before they die, and how they will leave their loved ones.

Nevertheless, many people die predictable deaths without the peace and comfort that the word *predictable* implies is possible. Death while receiving intensive medical care and while suffering from physical pain and other symptoms has been the norm since at least 1990 (Institute of Medicine, 1997; Singer et al., 2015), although most people say they want to die while experiencing pain and symptom control, socioemotional and religious or spiritual support, and dignity and quality of life (Meier et al., 2016; Steinhauser et al., 2000). Each chapter of this book has covered a facet of predictable death, shedding light on how it is historically novel, the current social responses to it in policy and practice, and the consequences of this set of responses. In this final chapter, I draw together those consequences to arrive at three broader directions for action to improve death and dying in the U.S. today.

Conclusion 1: Death is Predictable, so Health Care Professionals and Members of the General Public Alike Should Anticipate It

Before the epidemiological transition, death often occurred with little warning and was subject to little human control, but it was routine and familiar (Aries, 1982). People did not celebrate death, but it was a fact of existence. Now, the reverse is true: Three-quarters of deaths occur to adults over the age of 65, who die following a long chronic illness such as heart disease or cancer (Cubanski et al., 2016). At the same time, death is shocking and unacceptable in the minds of most people (Kaufman, 2015). Death quality would likely improve if the idea of death was more normalized, both within the health care system and more broadly across U.S. society.

In part, the normalization of death is something that should feature in standard medical training to a much greater extent than it does at present. There is a great deal of content available to teach. For example, there is a sizeable literature in communication and linguistics about topics such as how patients experience the receipt of a terminal diagnosis (Schaepe, 2011), the language that experienced doctors choose to tell patients that they will die soon (Broom et al., 2014; Gramling & Gramling, 2019), and why patients misunderstand their prognoses (Singh et al., 2017). Following a 2004 Institute of Medicine report on the importance of the behavioral and social sciences, federal grant money has become available to add these topics and other social scientific information to medical school curricula (Institute of Medicine, 2004).

If general medical education on death and dying is incomplete, specialty training in fields such as geriatrics and palliative medicine is even moreso. Referral to and enrollment in hospice depend in large part on health care professionals who recognize the approach of death and know about palliative care (Welch et al., 2008). Yet many medical students never care for a dying patient (Anderson et al., 2008). A minority completes a formal course or rotation in palliative care, with only 30% of U.S. medical schools requiring a course in palliative and hospice care, and only 19% requiring students to complete a palliative care or hospice rotation (Van Aalst-Cohen et al., 2008). Among schools that did mandate training in this subject, there was great variability in the specific requirements (Horowitz et al., 2013). Perhaps due to this low exposure, by the middle of 2019, only 8,200 U.S.

physicians had chosen to be board-certified as specialists in hospice and palliative care (American Academy of Hospice and Palliative Medicine, 2019). Experts estimate that the U.S. presently needs 11,000 such physicians to supply the population at a rate of 20 physicians per 100,000 older adults, and that by 2040, it will need 16,000 (Lupu et al., 2018).

Likewise, specialty certification in geriatrics has not kept pace with population aging. Approximately 30% of older adults should be under the care of geriatricians, who specialize in the "care of patients with multiple diseases; management and prevention of geriatric syndromes including frailty, falls, incontinence, disability, cognitive decline; prevention; prognosis; evaluating risk; and appropriately caring for older adults with different levels of health status" (Fried & Hall, 2008, p. 1792). In 2018, there were just under 7,000 physicians nationwide who were board-certified in geriatric medicine, and an additional 1,500 certified in geriatric psychiatry (American Board of Medical Specialties, 2018). Assuming that one geriatrician can care for 700 patients, the nation will require 33,000 certified geriatricians by 2025 (American Geriatrics Society, 2020).

However, medical students and health care professionals are not the only targets for normalizing death. The general public believes in the "rule of rescue," that doctors can save people from the disaster of death (Hetzler & Dugdale, 2018, p. 768). For example, cardiopulmonary resuscitation (CPR) saves fictional characters on medical dramas far more often than CPR is effective in reality (Portanova et al., 2015). People do not want to be burdened with death, and they expect their health care professionals to provide relief.

Since the 1960s, the death awareness movement has been a loosely organized group of largely grassroots efforts aimed at normalizing death in the general public (Doka, 2003). For example, the Death Café movement, developed in Switzerland and enjoying popularity in the U.S., is a community forum at which people gather with refreshments to reflect upon death, loss, and the meaning of life (Miles & Corr, 2017). The Project on Death in America and the non-profit organization called End Well are other recent, more activist-oriented efforts. At a larger scale, palliative care services in the UK are leading initiatives to create "compassionate communities" that better integrate hospices with other community services (Kellehear, 2013, p. 1071). For example, social contact between schoolchildren and hospice patients serves to teach school children about death and loss while lessening the isolation of dying people.

At a more individual level, there are efforts to increase rates of advance care planning: living wills, durable power of attorney appointments, and conversations with family and health care providers. However, over a quarter of adults aged 65 and older have done no advance care planning, and Spanish-speaking Latinos are especially unlikely to plan (Harrison et al., 2016). Advance care planning has a variety of limitations, but it does reduce hospitalizations in the last weeks of life, increase the use of hospice, result in less use of life-prolonging treatments, and aid the grief process for surviving loved ones (Brinkman-Stoppelenburg et al., 2014;

Khandelwal et al., 2015; Song et al., 2015; Teno et al., 2007). Key elements of doing it well include engaging in multiple types of planning, especially including conversations alongside legal plans, and repeating the process over time as families' composition, health care situations, and preferences change.

As of 2016, Medicare reimburses physicians for holding an advanced care planning discussion with a patient (Doukas, 2017). Some regional insurers have adopted more comprehensive programs. For example, the Respecting Choices program builds infrastructure in the health system to support advance care planning, such as certification for health care providers, includes community outreach and education, and yields significant evidence of its efficacy in multiple implementations (Briggs, 2013; Kirchhoff et al., 2012). At the level of the individual patient, organizations such as Aging with Dignity have created documents like Five Wishes, which is a living will written in layman's language, rather than legal language, in an effort to improve accessibility (Aging with Dignity, 2019). Furthermore, scholars continue to develop and rigorously test interventions to increase rates of planning (Song et al., 2015).

Conclusion 2: In the Absence of Thoughtfully-Designed Practices and Policies, Predictable Death Generates Social Disparities

Fundamental cause theory illustrates that the more humans learn about health and health behaviors, the more inequalities in health emerge. The reason is that people who have resources such as income are able to employ those resources to use the new health knowledge, while people who lack resources are unable to do so (Phelan & Link, 2005). For example, advance care planning is a health behavior that can help avert a typical, bad death. White non-Hispanic people who have high income and educational attainment complete advance care planning at high rates (Harrison et al., 2016). People who do not have these resources plan at much lower rates, and perhaps as a result, they experience deaths of poorer average quality.

This process of disparity generation – that knowledge exacerbates disparities – means that researchers, clinicians, and policymakers must think carefully about how to handle medical innovations. They are not a simple good that will make lives better in the absence of oversight, but rather may have unintended consequences in the form of health disparities. Disparities may appear in access, adoption, adherence, and/or effectiveness of the new health knowledge (Veinot et al., 2018). Even publication of health research can exacerbate disparities, because well-educated, wealthy people have first access to scholarly knowledge (Oster, 2018). Disparities may stabilize or even dissipate on their own with time, but typically only once no further gains can be made among advantaged people (Clouston et al., 2016).

Fortunately, the people who generate health care innovations are becoming aware of this problem. For example, people working in machine learning to create models to identify patients who are at risk of poor outcomes are increasingly taking note of the biases that can inadvertently enter the design process, as well as the ways fairness or equity can be built into the design (Rajkomar et al., 2018). The broad strategy that fundamental cause theory implies is that by design, health interventions should minimize the importance of an individual's resources (Phelan et al., 2010). Anything that happens automatically, rather than requiring a person's action, reduces disparities by reducing individuals' need to use resources. For example, far more people complete colorectal cancer screening when all are mailed a test kit than when people must make individual requests to be mailed a test kit (Mehta et al., 2018).

Notably, the people on the losing end of health disparities are not the people who have the power to create law or policy. For example, in 2018, 60.4% of Americans were non-Hispanic White (U.S. Census Bureau, 2018). Yet in 2019, 46 of the 50 states (92%) had a White non-Hispanic governor. These elected leaders do not represent the populace in a sociodemographic sense, nor are they elected by a sociodemographically representative body of the populace. The United States does not have mandatory voting laws, and non-Hispanic White, college-educated adults over the age of 60 have the highest turnout rates in elections (McDonald, 2019). These associations mirror socioeconomic disparities, and these effects may represent both the immediate and long-term effects of social exclusion: People who believe that their vote will have no effect choose not to vote (Fraga, 2016; Rocha et al., 2010). For example, Black voter turnout remains lowest in the parts of the country that had the highest prevalence of slavery (Acharya et al., 2016).

Of course, law and policy can represent the interests of disadvantaged populations even if lawmakers and voters themselves are not disadvantaged. However, the persistence of health inequalities suggests that some people are not represented. U.S. politicians recognize fundamental causes of disparity, but do not go so far as to advocate for the kinds of policies that might reduce disparities by redistributing resources (Lynch & Perera, 2017). They do not need to; the U.S. public is more tolerant of health disparities than is the public in other nations (Hero et al., 2017). Individuals hold stereotyped beliefs about the health behaviors of members of other sociodemographic groups, and many blame these health behaviors for health disparities (Gollust & Lynch, 2011). U.S. residents live in bubbles, socializing with others like themselves (DiPrete et al., 2011) and living and working with others like themselves (Krivo et al., 2013). These patterns lead to stereotyping, distrust of others, and unwillingness to act in the interests of others, even though greater equality in resources such as wealth would likely improve health for all Americans (Pickett & Wilkinson, 2015).

Conclusion 3: Bad Death is a Public Issue, not a Private Trouble

In the aftermath of a bad death, with care that did not enable the deceased person to fulfill their values and preferences for the end of life, families, and health care providers may look for someone to blame (Collins et al., 2009). Yet bad deaths are rarely the result of individual choices or particular personalities and relationships. Rather, bad deaths are a public issue: the result of the ways in which local, state, and national policies are structured (Mills, 1959). In this section, I make four recommendations for policies that could improve the predictable death in the U.S.

1. **Expand access to palliative care.** About half of people who die are receiving palliative care through the hospice benefit (National Hospice and Palliative Care Organization, 2017). Yet, to receive the hospice benefit, the patient have a physician's prognosis of six months or less to live, and agree to stop all curative treatments. Perhaps as a result of these strict limitations, over a quarter of hospice benefit recipients receive less than a week of palliative care (National Hospice and Palliative Care Organization, 2017). If Medicare paid for palliative care independent of the patient's prognosis and/or alongside curative care, the average quality of death in the U.S. would likely be better.

Since 2016, the Center for Medicare & Medicaid Innovation has been pilot testing a program reimbursing hospices $400 per patient per month to deliver palliative care services to patients who were continuing to receive curative care (Abt Associates, 2018). This program, called the Medicare Care Choices Model, is possible because of legislation in the 2010 Affordable Care Act that allows Medicare to test models of care that might reduce Medicare spending while improving patient outcomes (Centers for Medicare & Medicaid Services, 2018). A first cohort of patients began enrolling in 2016, and a second cohort began enrolling in 2018. The pilot is scheduled to run for five years, and 104 hospices across the country are participating.

An initial 2018 report provided two main findings (Abt Associates, 2018). First, a quarter of patients whose physicians referred them to the program chose to take the standard hospice benefit instead. This suggests that there is a group of hospice-eligible patients who are willing to end curative care, but lack the information or resources to enroll in hospice without assistance from the health care system. Second, 14% of patients who died in the first year died while still receiving pilot program services, while 83% died after having transitioned to the standard hospice benefit without curative care. Those who entered standard hospice received those services for an average of 1 month before they died. This is a good rate of success, and hospice staff felt that the program was beneficial because it allowed patients and families to develop a relationship with hospice before the patient's death was imminent.

2. **Create migration mechanisms for paid care workers.** Paid care workers are in high demand, yet care jobs do not carry the salaries or benefits that employers usually use to entice workers when competing to hire them. This situation has produced inadequacies in care quality for people dying predictable deaths (Graham, 2017). These inadequacies are likely to become worse as the demand for workers further outstrips the supply of U.S. women in midlife, who are most likely to take care jobs (Dawson, 2016).

Given the high demand for care workers, one set of solutions is to create mechanisms for migrants to legally enter the U.S. to do such work. Current work visa mechanisms favor migrants with high levels of education who have the unique skills to perform specialized jobs, and so few are issued to care workers. Other highly developed nations with aging populations are actively exploring novel migration options for care workers. Some countries offer care worker incentives within their temporary visa programs. For example, Spain and Italy have relaxed rules requiring a new work permit application if a care worker changes employers within the industry, and Austria and Italy have exempted care workers from counting towards quotas on immigration of people from outside the European Union (Fujisawa & Colombo, 2009).

Some countries have also experimented with their programs for permanent migration. For example, Japan has bilateral agreements with Indonesia, the Philippines, and Vietnam, where citizens of those countries can migrate to Japan indefinitely to take care jobs, provided that they demonstrate language proficiency and pass an exam (Stone, 2016). Such an agreement between the U.S. and the nations where care workers most commonly come from – Mexico, the Philippines, and Jamaica – could reduce the number of undocumented migrants in care work (Chen et al., 2013).

Until the end of 2019, Canada ran the Live-In Caregiver program, which was an employer-specific work permit that offered the opportunity to apply for permanent resident status after 2 years of doing care work in the country (Canadian Immigration Law Firm, 2017). The program's popularity was in part why it ended, because of the backlog of applications. The country began separate programs for child care and for care for people with high medical need that promise to process applications within 6 months (Canadian Immigration Law Firm, 2017). The United Kingdom also ran a successful program that helped care workers to immigrate, but has subsequently reduced the size of the program and tightened the eligibility requirements for would-be workers (Spencer et al., 2010).

3. **Compensate unpaid family care work.** The belief that care work is a family responsibility is one of the factors that has prevented the crisis in care work from becoming a larger political issue (Levitsky, 2014). Each year, over 40 million unpaid care workers deliver 37 billion hours of care to adult care recipients (Reinhard et al., 2015). A third of these care workers have been providing care for more than five years, and an additional 15% have been providing care for more than ten years (National Academies of Sciences, Engineering, and Medicine et al., 2016). The average unpaid care worker spends 20% of his or her annual income on care, when the money could be going to the care worker's own retirement savings and thus preventing the care worker's own poverty in later life (Rainville et al., 2016; Wakabayashi & Donato, 2006).

Scholars have formulated proposals for Social Security to compensate unpaid care workers for the years of income they forgo. A comprehensive change would be to establish a minimum benefit that is adequate for living, regardless of one's work history (Herd et al., 2018). A more modest proposal, but one that has gained somewhat more political traction, is to give both men and women Social Security credit for years of family service (Estes et al., 2012). Beginning in the 1990s and every year since 2014, care provider credit acts have been introduced in Congress (Rocco, 2017). The 2019 bill proposed to credit up to five years of care on a sliding scale for people currently earning less than average wages, with the maximum credit for people not in the paid labor force (C. Murphy, 2019). These bills have gone no further than introduction, despite bipartisan support. In contrast, almost all European Union countries incorporate care provider credits for parents into their government pension programs, and a smaller number of countries also credit eldercare. Germany, for example, calculates a credit based on hours worked per week in the paid labor force, hours of unpaid care provided, and the care recipient's level of disability (Jankowski, 2011).

One alternative to Social Security reform is to pay currently unpaid care workers. Medicaid waivers programs in all states allow benefit recipients to self-direct their care rather than have the state administer it (Centers for Medicare & Medicaid Services, 2020). In self-direction programs, recipients can use Medicaid money for a variety of purposes, including hiring family members as care providers in some circumstances. These programs have good outcomes for patients and care workers alike, and they save Medicaid money (Newcomer et al., 2012; Simon-Rusinowitz et al., 2005). The programs have not been wildly popular, however, in part because family members are often reluctant to accept the funds (Stacey & Ayers, 2012).

4. **Create public health insurance for Americans of all ages.** Medicare covers almost all Americans who are over the age of 65. But in 2018, 10.4% of Americans who were younger than 65 had no health insurance (Tolbert et al., 2019). Compared to only 9% of insured adults, 28% of uninsured adults reported delaying or going without medical care due to the cost (Claxton et al., 2019). Some of these uninsured people will not survive to the Medicare eligibility age, and if they do, Medicare will not be able to fully compensate for years of foregone or inadequate care (Woolhandler & Himmelstein, 2017). Thus health care law for younger Americans will have consequences for the likelihood of good death – as well as for public Medicare and Medicaid spending – in future decades.

One estimate is that half of uninsured people qualify for Medicaid or for a public subsidy to purchase insurance (Gunja & Collins, 2019). These people may need assistance navigating complex application and enrollment procedures, or they may benefit from reforms that subsidize existing programs more generously. But these people, in addition to the remaining half of uninsured people, may benefit as well programs that are common elsewhere but dramatically new to the United States. A majority of Americans favors a public single-payer system to the current system, and likewise, a majority of Americans favors a public insurance alternative within the current system (Lopes et al., 2020). Nations such as the United Kingdom have the former type of system, while nations such as Germany have the latter type of system. Either of these systems could take many different forms (Neuman et al., 2019). Experts estimate that even a single-payer system, which the public widely believes to be extremely expensive, would in fact reduce national health care expenditures by 13% (Galvani et al., 2020; Himmelstein et al., 2020). Regardless of specific form, any policy that reduces premature mortality and functional disability among younger adults is likely to result in more, and better, predictable deaths in old age.

Last Words

Improved standards of living and public health initiatives in the U.S. and elsewhere brought about a transition from high rates of death from infectious diseases to low rates of death from chronic, non-communicable illnesses. Most Americans can now expect to live to old age, and this expectation has made deaths, as well as entire lives, more predictable. However, the U.S. has largely failed to restructure public policy to be in accord with predictable deaths. As a result, most deaths include multiple hospitalizations, invasive and intensive treatments, and a high symptom burden. There is very little policy to support long-term care for people with chronic, disabling illnesses, leaving dying people and those who care for them in poverty and social isolation. Law to protect patients' personal autonomy is out of step with clinical realities. To the extent that solutions exist, they are aimed at individuals rather than communities, and are primarily accessible to people who enjoy social advantages such as White race/ethnicity and educational attainment. Nothing less than a renaissance in public policy is necessary to realize the possibilities inherent in the era of predictable death.

References

Abt Associates. (2018). *Evaluation of the Medicare Care Choices Model Annual Report #1*. Centers for Medicare & Medicaid Services. https://innovation.cms.gov/initiatives/Medicare-Care-Choices/.

Acharya, A., Blackwell, M., & Sen, M. (2016). *A culture of disenfranchisement: How American slavery continues to affect voting behavior*. Harvard University. https://scholar.harvard.edu/msen/slavery-voting-behavior.

Aging with Dignity. (2019). *Five Wishes*. https://fivewishes.org/.

American Academy of Hospice and Palliative Medicine. (2019). *Workforce data and reports*. http://aahpm.org/career/workforce-study#HPMphysicians.

American Board of Medical Specialties. (2018). *ABMS board certification report (2017–2018)* (p. 62). www.abms.org/media/194885/abms-board-certification-report-2017-2018.pdf.

American Geriatrics Society. (2020). *Geriatrics workforce by the numbers*. www.americangeriatrics.org/geriatrics-profession/about-geriatrics/geriatrics-workforce-numbers.

Anderson, W. G., Williams, J. E., Bost, J. E., & Barnard, D. (2008). Exposure to death is associated with positive attitudes and higher knowledge about end-of-life care in graduating medical students. *Journal of Palliative Medicine*, *11*(9), 1227–1233. https://doi.org/10.1089/jpm.2008.0058.

Aries, P. (1982). *The hour of our death*. Penguin Random House.

Arnett, J. J. (2000). Emerging adulthood: A theory of development from the late teens through the twenties. *American Psychologist, 55*(5), 469–480. https://doi.org/10.1037/0003-066X.55.5.469.

Briggs, L. A. (2013). Respecting Choices: An evidence-based advance care planning program with proven success and replication. In L. Rogne & S. L. McCune (Eds.), *Advance Care Planning: Communicating About Matters of Life and Death*. Springer Publishing Company.

Brinkman-Stoppelenburg, A., Rietjens, J. A., & van der Heide, A. (2014). The effects of advance care planning on end-of-life care: A systematic review. *Palliative Medicine, 28*(8), 1000–1025. https://doi.org/10.1177/0269216314526272.

Broom, A., Kirby, E., Good, P., Wootton, J., & Adams, J. (2014). The troubles of telling: Managing communication about the end of life. *Qualitative Health Research, 24*(2), 151–162. https://doi.org/10.1177/1049732313519709.

Canadian Immigration Law Firm. (2017, May 26). *Canada Live In Caregiver Program 2017 program update*. Canadim. www.canadim.com/blog/live-in-caregiver-2017-update/.

Carr, D., & Luth, E. A. (2019). Well-being at the end of life. *Annual Review of Sociology, 45*(1), 515–534. https://doi.org/10.1146/annurev-soc-073018-022524.

Centers for Medicare & Medicaid Services. (2018). *Medicare Care Choices Model: Frequently asked questions*. https://cmmicoordinator.survey.fm/was-this-helpful?iframe=https%3A%2F%2Finnovation.cms.gov%2Finitiatives%2FMedicare-Care-Choices%2Ffaq.html&ft=1.

Centers for Medicare & Medicaid Services. (2020). *Self-directed services*. www.medicaid.gov/medicaid/long-term-services-supports/self-directed-services/index.html.

Chen, P. G., Auerbach, D. I., Muench, U., Curry, L. A., & Bradley, E. H. (2013). Policy solutions to address the foreign-educated and foreign-born health care workforce in the United States. *Health Affairs, 32*(11), 1906–1913. https://doi.org/10.1377/hlthaff.2013.0576.

Cicirelli, V. G. (2011). Elders' attitudes toward extending the healthy life span. *Journal of Aging Studies, 25*(2), 84–93. https://doi.org/10.1016/j.jaging.2010.08.011.

Claxton, G., Sawyer, B., & Cox, C. (2019). How does cost affect access to care? *Peterson-Kaiser Health System Tracker*. www.healthsystemtracker.org/chart-collection/cost-affect-access-care/.

Clouston, S. A. P., Rubin, M. S., Phelan, J. C., & Link, B. G. (2016). A social history of disease: Contextualizing the rise and fall of social inequalities in cause-specific mortality. *Demography, 53*(5), 1631–1656. https://doi.org/10.1007/s13524-016-0495-5.

Collins, M. E., Block, S. D., Arnold, R. M., & Christakis, N. A. (2009). On the prospects for a blame-free medical culture. *Social Science & Medicine, 69*(9), 1287–1290. https://doi.org/10.1016/j.socscimed.2009.08.033.

Cubanski, J., Neuman, T., Griffin, S., & Damico, A. (2016). *Medicare spending at the end of life: A snapshot of beneficiaries who died in 2014 and the cost of their care*. Henry J. Kaiser Family Foundation. www.kff.org/medicare/issue-brief/medicare-spending-at-the-end-of-life/.

Dawson, S. L. (2016). The direct care workforce – Raising the floor of job quality. *Generations, 40*(1), 38–46.

DiPrete, T. A., Gelman, A., McCormick, T., Teitler, J., & Zheng, T. (2011). Segregation in social networks based on acquaintanceship and trust. *American Journal of Sociology, 116*(4), 1234–1283. https://doi.org/10.1086/659100.

Doka, K. J. (2003). The death awareness movement: Description, history, and analysis. In *Handbook of Death & Dying* (pp. 50–56). SAGE Publications, Inc. https://doi.org/10.4135/9781412914291.

Doukas, D. J. (2017). Advance care planning: Counseling in the wake of CMS reform. *Archives of Family Medicine and General Practice, 1*(2), 48–53. https://doi.org/10.36959/577/480.

Ekerdt, D. J., Koss, C. S., Li, A., Münch, A., Lessenich, S., & Fung, H. H. (2017). Is longevity a value for older adults? *Journal of Aging Studies, 43*, 46–52. https://doi.org/10.1016/j.jaging.2017.10.002.

Estes, C., O'Neill, T., & Hartmann, H. (2012). *Breaking the Social Security glass ceiling: A proposal to modernize women's benefits*. Institute for Women's Policy Research. https://iwpr.org/publications/breaking-the-social-security-glass-ceiling-a-proposal-to-modernize-womens-benefits/.

Fraga, B. L. (2016). Candidates or districts? Reevaluating the role of race in voter turnout. *American Journal of Political Science, 60*(1), 97–122. https://doi.org/10.1111/ajps.12172.

Fried, L. P., & Hall, W. J. (2008). Leading on behalf of an aging society. *Journal of the American Geriatrics Society, 56*(10), 1791–1795. https://doi.org/10.1111/j.1532-5415.2008.01939.x.

Fujisawa, R., & Colombo, F. (2009). *The long-term care workforce: Overview and strategies to adapt supply to a growing demand* (Health Working Papers No. 44). OECD. www.oecd-ilibrary.org/social-issues-migration-health/the-long-term-care-workforce-overview-and-strategies-to-adapt-supply-to-a-growing-demand_225350638472.

Galvani, A. P., Parpia, A. S., Foster, E. M., Singer, B. H., & Fitzpatrick, M. C. (2020). Improving the prognosis of health care in the USA. *The Lancet, 395*(10223), 524–533. https://doi.org/10.1016/S0140-6736(19)33019-3.

Gollust, S. E., & Lynch, J. (2011). Who deserves health care? The effects of causal attributions and group cues on public attitudes about responsibility for health care costs. *Journal of Health Politics, Policy and Law, 36*(6), 1061–1095. https://doi.org/10.1215/03616878-1460578.

Graham, J. (2017). Severe shortage of home health workers robs thousands of proper care. *Kaiser Health News*. https://khn.org/news/severe-shortage-of-home-health-workers-robs-thousands-of-proper-care/.

Gramling, D., & Gramling, R. (2019). *Palliative care conversations: Clinical and applied linguistic perspectives*. Walter de Gruyter.

Gunja, M. Z., & Collins, S. R. (2019). *Who are the remaining uninsured, and why do they lack coverage?* Commonwealth Fund. https://doi.org/10.26099/h0xy-az24.

Harrison, K. L., Adrion, E. R., Ritchie, C. S., Sudore, R. L., & Smith, A. K. (2016). Low completion and disparities in advance care planning activities among older Medicare beneficiaries. *Journal of the American Medical Association Internal Medicine, 176*(12), 1872–1875. https://doi.org/10.1001/jamainternmed.2016.6751.

Herd, P., Favreault, M., Harrington Meyer, M., & Smeeding, T. M. (2018). A targeted minimum benefit plan: A new proposal to reduce poverty among older Social Security recipients a targeted minimum benefit plan. *Public Policy & Aging Report, 28*(S1), S35–S40. https://doi.org/10.1093/ppar/pry022.

Hero, J. O., Zaslavsky, A. M., & Blendon, R. J. (2017). The United States leads other nations in differences by income in perceptions of health and health care. *Health Affairs, 36*(6), 1032–1040. https://doi.org/10.1377/hlthaff.2017.0006.

Hetzler, P. T., & Dugdale, L. S. (2018). How do medicalization and rescue fantasy prevent healthy dying? *AMA Journal of Ethics, 20*(8), 766–773. https://doi.org/10.1001/amajethics.2018.766.

Himmelstein, D. U., Campbell, T., & Woolhandler, S. (2020). Health care administrative costs in the United States and Canada, 2017. *Annals of Internal Medicine, 172*(2), 134. https://doi.org/10.7326/M19-2818.

Horowitz, R., Gramling, R., & Quill, T. E. (2013). Palliative care education in U.S. medical schools. *Medical Education, 48*(1), 59–66. https://doi.org/10.1111/medu.12292.

Institute of Medicine. (1997). *Approaching death: Improving care at the end of life* (M. J. Field & C. K. Cassel, Eds.). National Academies Press.

Institute of Medicine. (2004). *Improving medical education: Enhancing the behavioral and social science content of medical school curricula*. http://nationalacademies.org/hmd/Reports/2004/Improving-Medical-Education-Enhancing-the-Behavioral-and-Social-Science-Content-of-Medical-School-Curricula.aspx.

Jankowski, J. (2011). Caregiver credits in France, Germany, and Sweden: Lessons for the United States. *Social Security Bulletin, 71*(4), 61–76.

Kahana, E., Kahana, B., & Zhang, J. (2005). Motivational antecedents of preventive proactivity in late life: Linking future orientation and exercise. *Motivation and Emotion, 29*(4), 438–459. https://doi.org/10.1007/s11031-006-9012-2.

Kaufman, S. R. (2015). *Ordinary medicine*. Duke University Press.

Kellehear, A. (2013). Compassionate communities: End-of-life care as everyone's responsibility. *QJM: An International Journal of Medicine, 106*(12), 1071–1075. https://doi.org/10.1093/qjmed/hct200.

Khandelwal, N., Kross, E. K., Engelberg, R. A., Coe, N. B., Long, A. C., & Curtis, J. R. (2015). Estimating the effect of palliative care interventions and advance care planning on ICU utilization: A systematic review. *Critical Care Medicine, 43*(5), 1102–1111. https://doi.org/10.1097/CCM.0000000000000852.

Kirchhoff, K. T., Hammes, B. J., Kehl, K. A., Briggs, L. A., & Brown, R. L. (2012). Effect of a Disease-Specific Advance Care Planning Intervention on End-of-Life Care. *Journal of the American Geriatrics Society, 60*(5), 946–950. https://doi.org/10.1111/j.1532-5415.2012.03917.x.

Kotter-Grühn, D., Grühn, D., & Smith, J. (2010). Predicting one's own death: The relationship between subjective and objective nearness to death in very old age. *European Journal of Ageing, 7*(4), 293–300. https://doi.org/10.1007/s10433-010-0165-1.

Krivo, L. J., Washington, H. M., Peterson, R. D., Browning, C. R., Calder, C. A., & Kwan, M.-P. (2013). Social isolation of disadvantage and advantage: The reproduction of inequality in urban space. *Social Forces, 92*(1), 141–164. https://doi.org/10.1093/sf/sot043.

Levitsky, S. R. (2014). *Caring for our own: Why there is no political demand for new American social welfare rights*. Oxford University Press.

Levy, B. R., Slade, M. D., Murphy, T. E., & Gill, T. M. (2012). Association between positive age stereotypes and recovery from disability in older persons. *Journal of the American Medical Association, 308*(19), 1972–1973. https://doi.org/10.1001/jama.2012.14541.

Lopes, L., Hamel, L., Kearney, A., & Brodie, M. (2020, January 30). Medicare-for-all, public option, health care legislation and court actions. *The Henry J. Kaiser Family Foundation*. www.kff.org/health-reform/poll-finding/kff-health-tracking-poll-january-2020/.

Lupu, D., Quigley, L., Mehfoud, N., & Salsberg, E. S. (2018). The growing demand for hospice and palliative medicine physicians: Will the supply keep up? *Journal of Pain and Symptom Management, 55*(4), 1216–1223. https://doi.org/10.1016/j.jpainsymman.2018.01.011.

Lynch, J. F., & Perera, I. M. (2017). Framing health equity: U.S. health disparities in comparative perspective. *Journal of Health Politics, Policy and Law, 42*(5), 803–839. https://doi.org/10.1215/03616878-3940450.

McDonald, M. P. (2019). *Voter turnout demographics*. United States Elections Project. www.electproject.org/home/voter-turnout/demographics.

Mehta, S., Khan, T., Guerra, C., Reitz, C., McAuliffe, T., Volpp, K., Asch, D., & Doubeni, C. (2018). A randomized controlled trial of opt-in versus opt-out colorectal cancer screening outreach. *American Journal of Gastroenterology, 113*(12), 1848–1854. https://doi.org/10.1038/s41395-018-0151-3.

Meier, E. A., Gallegos, J. V., Thomas, L. P. M., Depp, C. A., Irwin, S. A., & Jeste, D.V. (2016). Defining a good death (successful dying): Literature review and a call for research and public dialogue. *The American Journal of Geriatric Psychiatry, 24*(4), 261–271. https://doi.org/10.1016/j.jagp.2016.01.135.

Miles, L., & Corr, C.A. (2017). Death cafe: What is it and what we can learn from it. *OMEGA – Journal of Death and Dying, 75*(2), 151–165. https://doi.org/10.1177/0030222815612602.

Mills, C.W. (1959). *The sociological imagination*. Oxford University Press.

Mirowsky, J. (1997). Age, subjective life expectancy, and the sense of control: The horizon hypothesis. *The Journals of Gerontology: Series B, 52B*(3), S125–S134. https://doi.org/10.1093/geronb/52B.3.S125.

Murphy, C. (2019, July 30). *Social Security Caregiver Credit Act of 2019* [Webpage]. www.congress.gov/bill/116th-congress/senate-bill/2317/text.

Murphy, S. L., Xu, J., Kochanek, K., & Arias, E. (2018). *Mortality in the United States, 2017* (NCHS Data Brief No. 328). National Center for Health Statistics. www.cdc.gov/nchs/products/databriefs/db328.htm.

National Academies of Sciences, Engineering, and Medicine, Eden, J., Adults, C. on F. C. for O., Services, B. on H. C., Division, H. and M., & National Academies of Sciences, E. (2016). *Families caring for an aging America*. National Academies Press. www.ncbi.nlm.nih.gov/books/NBK396409/.

National Hospice and Palliative Care Organization. (2017). *Facts and figures: Hospice care in America*. www.nhpco.org/sites/default/files/public/Statistics_Research/2017_Facts_Figures.pdf.

Neuman, T., Pollitz, K., Tolbert, J., Rudowitz, R., & Koma, W. (2019, December 18). 10 key questions on public option proposals. *The Henry J. Kaiser Family Foundation*. www.kff.org/health-reform/issue-brief/10-key-questions-on-public-option-proposals/.

Newcomer, R. J., Kang, T., & Doty, P. (2012). Allowing spouses to be paid personal care providers: Spouse availability and effects on medicaid-funded service use and expenditures. *The Gerontologist, 52*(4), 517–530. https://doi.org/10.1093/geront/gnr102.

Oster, E. (2018). *Behavioral feedback: Do individual choices influence scientific results?* [National Bureau of Economic Research Working Paper]. National Bureau of Economic Research. https://doi.org/10.3386/w25225.

Phelan, J. C., & Link, B. G. (2005). Controlling disease and creating disparities: A fundamental cause perspective. *The Journals of Gerontology: Series B, 60*(Special_Issue_2), S27–S33. https://doi.org/10.1093/geronb/60.Special_Issue_2.S27.

Phelan, J. C., Link, B. G., & Tehranifar, P. (2010). Social conditions as fundamental causes of health inequalities: Theory, evidence, and policy implications. *Journal of Health and Social Behavior, 51*(1_suppl), S28–S40. https://doi.org/10.1177/0022146510383498.

Pickett, K. E., & Wilkinson, R. G. (2015). Income inequality and health: A causal review. *Social Science & Medicine, 128*, 316–326. https://doi.org/10.1016/j.socscimed.2014.12.031.

Portanova, J., Irvine, K., Yi, J. Y., & Enguidanos, S. (2015). It isn't like this on TV: Revisiting CPR survival rates depicted on popular TV shows. *Resuscitation, 96*, 148–150. https://doi.org/10.1016/j.resuscitation.2015.08.002.

Rainville, C., Skufca, L., & Mehegan, L. (2016). *Family caregivers cost survey: What they spend & what they sacrifice*. AARP. www.aarp.org/research/topics/care/info-2016/family-caregivers-cost-survey.html?CMP=RDRCT-PPI-CAREGIVING-102416.

Rajkomar, A., Hardt, M., Howell, M. D., Corrado, G., & Chin, M. H. (2018). Ensuring fairness in machine learning to advance health equity. *Annals of Internal Medicine, 169*(12), 866. https://doi.org/10.7326/M18-1990.

Reinhard, S., Feinberg, L. F., Choula, R., & Houser, A. (2015). *Valuing the invaluable: 2015 update.* AARP. www.aarp.org/ppi/info-2015/valuing-the-invaluable-2015-update.html.

Rocco, P. (2017). Informal caregiving and the politics of policy drift in the United States. *Journal of Aging & Social Policy, 29*(5), 413–432. https://doi.org/10.1080/08959420.2017.1280748.

Rocha, R. R., Tolbert, C. J., Bowen, D. C., & Clark, C. J. (2010). Race and turnout: Does descriptive representation in state legislatures increase minority voting? *Political Research Quarterly, 63*(4), 890–907. https://doi.org/10.1177/1065912910376388.

Schaepe, K. S. (2011). Bad news and first impressions: Patient and family caregiver accounts of learning the cancer diagnosis. *Social Science & Medicine, 73*(6), 912–921. https://doi.org/10.1016/j.socscimed.2011.06.038.

Simon-Rusinowitz, L., Mahoney, K. J., Loughlin, D. M., & Sadler, M. D. (2005). Paying family caregivers: An effective policy option in the Arkansas Cash and Counseling Demonstration and Evaluation. *Marriage & Family Review, 37*(1–2), 83–105. https://doi.org/10.1300/J002v37n01_07.

Singer, A. E., Meeker, D., Teno, J. M., Lynn, J., Lunney, J. R., & Lorenz, K. A. (2015). Symptom trends in the last year of life from 1998 to 2010: A cohort study. *Annals of Internal Medicine, 162*(3), 175. https://doi.org/10.7326/M13-1609.

Singh, S., Cortez, D., Maynard, D., Cleary, J. F., DuBenske, L., & Campbell, T. C. (2017). Characterizing the nature of scan results discussions: Insights into why patients misunderstand their prognosis. *Journal of Oncology Practice, 13*(3), e231–e239. https://doi.org/10.1200/JOP.2016.014621.

Song, M.-K., Ward, S. E., Fine, J. P., Hanson, L. C., Lin, F.-C., Hladik, G. A., Hamilton, J. B., & Bridgman, J. C. (2015). Advance care planning and end-of-life decision making in dialysis: A randomized controlled trial targeting patients and their surrogates. *American Journal of Kidney Diseases, 66*(5), 813–822. https://doi.org/10.1053/j.ajkd.2015.05.018.

Spencer, S., Martin, S., Bourgeault, I. L., & O'Shea, E. (2010). *The role of migrant care workers in ageing societies: Report on research findings in the United Kingdom, Ireland, Canada and the United States* (Migration Research Series No. 41; p. 84). International Organization for Migration.

Stacey, C. L., & Ayers, L. L. (2012). Caught between love and money: The experiences of paid family caregivers. *Qualitative Sociology, 35*(1), 47–64. https://doi.org/10.1007/s11133-011-9210-4.

Steinhauser, K. E., Clipp, E. C., McNeilly, M., Christakis, N. A., McIntyre, L. M., & Tulsky, J. A. (2000). In search of a good death: Observations of patients, families, and providers. *Annals of Internal Medicine, 132*(10), 825. https://doi.org/10.7326/0003-4819-132-10-200005160-00011.

Stone, R. I. (2016). The migrant direct care workforce: An international perspective. *Generations, 40*(1), 99–105.

Swisher, R. R., & Warner, T. D. (2013). If they grow up: Exploring the neighborhood context of adolescent and young adult survival expectations. *Journal of Research on Adolescence, 23*(4), 678–694. https://doi.org/10.1111/jora.12027.

Teno, J. M., Gruneir, A., Schwartz, Z., Nanda, A., & Wetle, T. (2007). Association between advance directives and quality of end-of-life care: A national study. *Journal of the American Geriatrics Society, 55*(2), 189–194. https://doi.org/10.1111/j.1532-5415.2007.01045.x.

Tolbert, J., Orgera, K., Singer, N., & Damico, A. (2019). *Key facts about the uninsured population*. Kaiser Family Foundation. www.kff.org/uninsured/fact-sheet/key-facts-about-the-uninsured-population/.

U.S. Census Bureau. (2018). *QuickFacts: United States*. www.census.gov/quickfacts/fact/table/US/PST045218.

Van Aalst-Cohen, E. S., Riggs, R., & Byock, I. R. (2008). Palliative care in medical school curricula: A survey of United States medical schools. *Journal of Palliative Medicine, 11*(9), 1200–1202. https://doi.org/10.1089/jpm.2008.0118.

Veinot, T. C., Mitchell, H., & Ancker, J. S. (2018). Good intentions are not enough: How informatics interventions can worsen inequality. *Journal of the American Medical Informatics Association, 25*(8), 1080–1088. https://doi.org/10.1093/jamia/ocy052.

Wakabayashi, C., & Donato, K. M. (2006). Does caregiving increase poverty among women in later life? Evidence from the Health and Retirement survey. *Journal of Health and Social Behavior, 47*(3), 258–274. https://doi.org/10.1177/002214650604700305.

Welch, L. C., Miller, S. C., Martin, E. W., & Nanda, A. (2008). Referral and timing of referral to hospice care in nursing homes: The significant role of staff members. *The Gerontologist, 48*(4), 477–484. https://doi.org/10.1093/geront/48.4.477.

Woolhandler, S., & Himmelstein, D. U. (2017). The relationship of health insurance and mortality: Is lack of insurance deadly? *Annals of Internal Medicine, 167*(6), 424. https://doi.org/10.7326/M17-1403.

INDEX

Page numbers in **bold** denote tables.